To
DAD,
on HIS
91st B'day!
Lots of Love,
Barbara
Sept 9, 2023

# THE Blue Zones

## Secrets for Living Longer

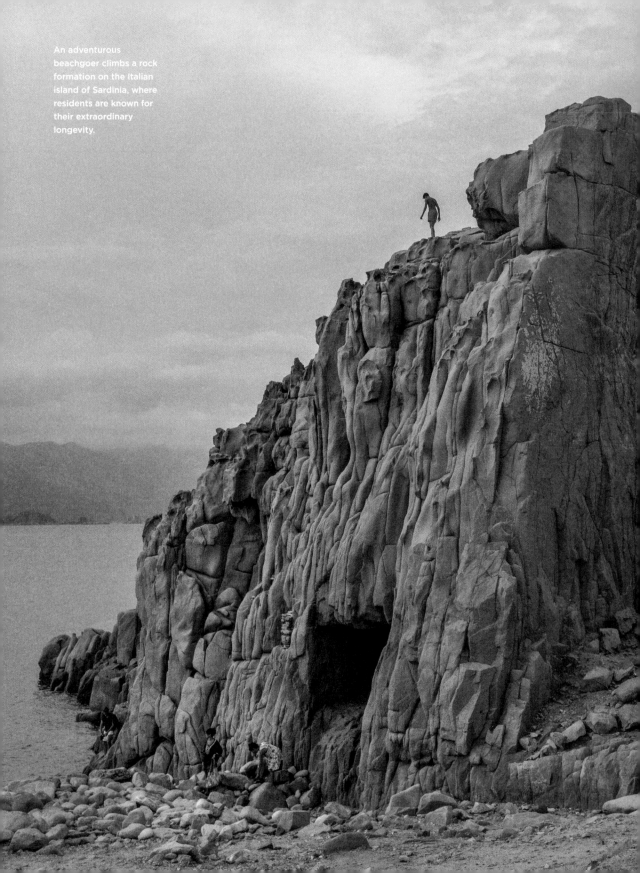

An adventurous beachgoer climbs a rock formation on the Italian island of Sardinia, where residents are known for their extraordinary longevity.

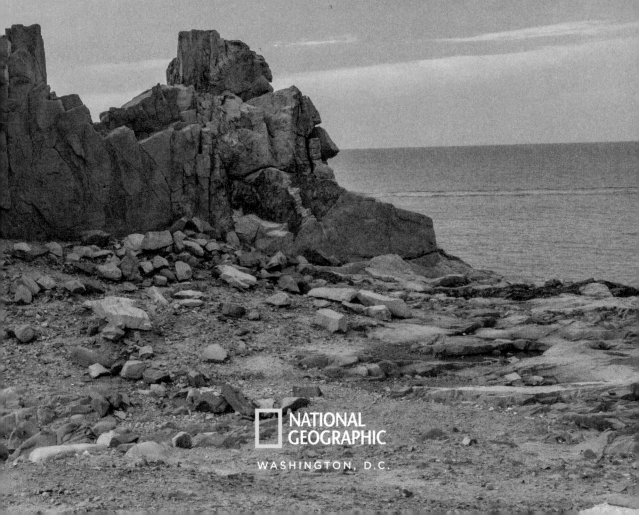

# THE Blue Zones
## Secrets for Living Longer
### Lessons From the Healthiest Places on Earth

**DAN BUETTNER**

NATIONAL GEOGRAPHIC

WASHINGTON, D.C.

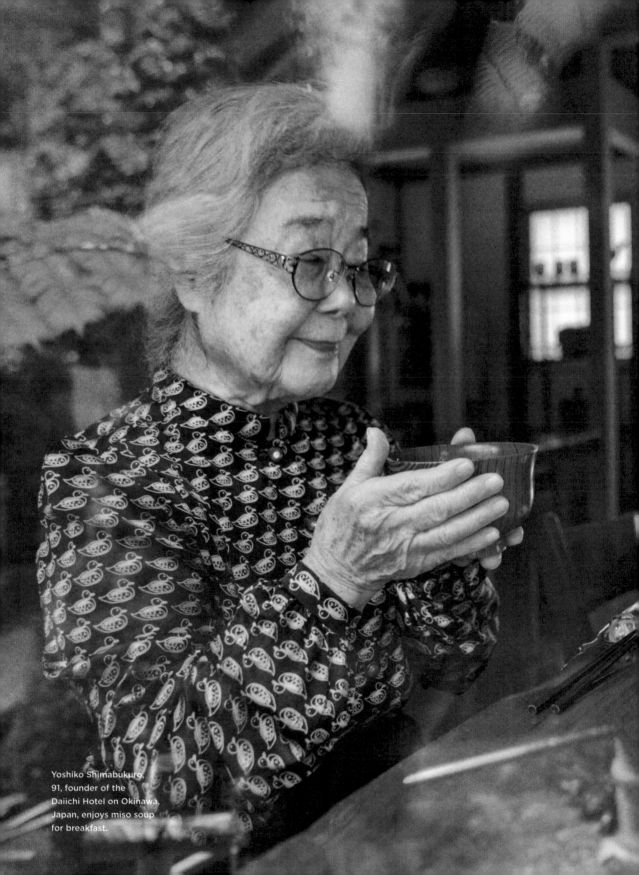

Yoshiko Shimabukuro, 91, founder of the Daiichi Hotel on Okinawa, Japan, enjoys miso soup for breakfast.

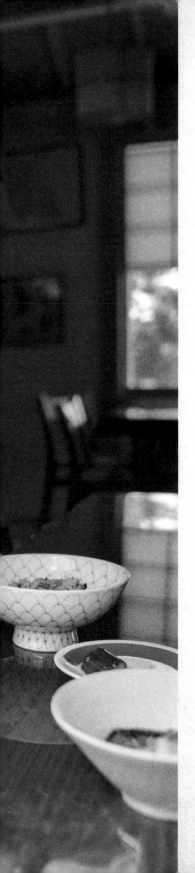

# Contents

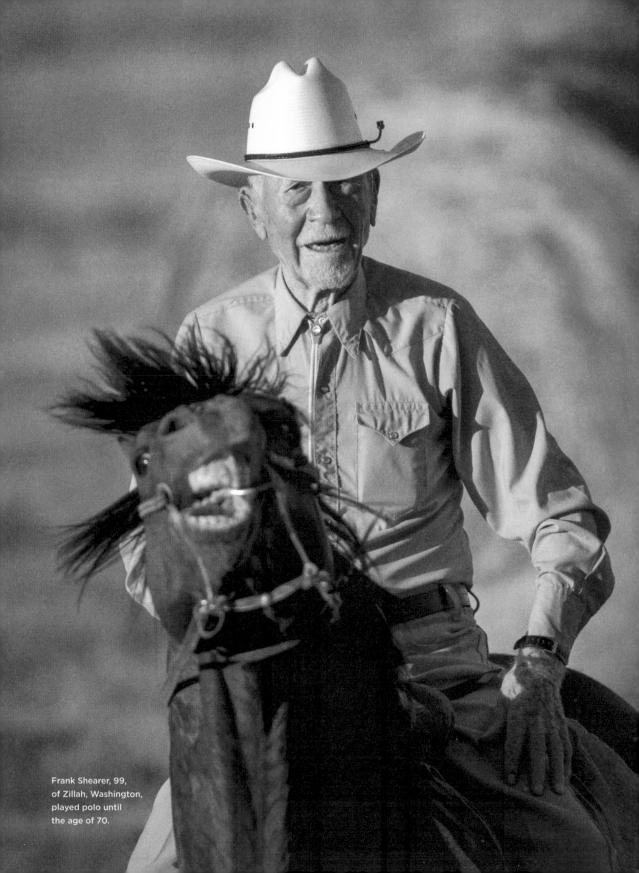

Frank Shearer, 99,
of Zillah, Washington,
played polo until
the age of 70.

# The Birth
# of the Blue Zones

Most of what we think will help us live longer and healthier is misguided or just plain wrong. It's common sense to get on a diet regimen, join a gym, and get our vitamins, right? Let's take a closer look.

In 2021, Americans spent more than $151 billion on vitamins and supplements (vitamin C, omega-3s, multivitamins, and the like). But the biggest, most dependable studies show that people who take supplements actually live shorter lives than people who don't. Americans spent another $21 billion or so on protein supplements. But according to the Centers for Disease Control and Prevention, the average American gets about twice as much protein as they need. In fact, no supplement, pill, hormone, or vitamin has ever proved to extend life expectancy in humans.

The concept of exercise—physical effort carried out to sustain or improve health and fitness—has been around in the United States since at least 1820. It's a nice idea to stay fit. And indeed, people who stay physically active have about a 30 percent lower chance of dying in any given year than people who aren't active. But despite the $160 billion per year Americans spend on trying to exercise, only about a fifth of all adults get the minimum recommended amount of vigorous activity (about 11 minutes a day). That means exercise is not working for more than 200 million Americans.

Similarly, diets are a well-intentioned but colossally ineffective approach to staying healthy and living longer. They fail for almost everyone almost all the time. Take 100 people who resolve to diet on New Year's Eve and by January 19 most will have abandoned the effort. By August only 10 percent will still be trying to eat better, and within two years the success rate will be under 5 percent. If your financial planner returned those yields, you'd fire him. Yet we spend $200 billion a year thinking that *this time* the diet will work.

So, if the most common approaches to better health and longevity don't work, what does?

In the early 2000s I set out to reverse engineer longevity. Under the mentorship of Dr. Ancel Keys and Dr. Robert Kane of the University of Minnesota's School of Public Health, I relied on two assumptions: First, genes have relatively little impact on how long we live. A Danish twin study in 1996 found that longevity is only mildly heritable, accounting for only about a fourth of the health differences among people. The rest is largely driven by our environment. Second, in those places around the world where people are living longer, they're doing something right. If I could find demographically confirmed areas where people were living the longest and identify the lifestyle commonalities of those regions, I might discern some clues.

Rather than searching for answers in a test tube or a petri dish, I looked for them among populations that have achieved what we want—long, healthy lives and sharp brains until the end. The idea garnered a grant from the National Institutes on Aging and a *National Geographic* assignment.

> RATHER THAN SEARCHING FOR ANSWERS IN A TEST TUBE OR A PETRI DISH, I LOOKED FOR THEM AMONG POPULATIONS THAT HAVE ACHIEVED WHAT WE WANT— LONG, HEALTHY LIVES AND SHARP BRAINS UNTIL THE END.

Armed with a plan, I began a worldwide search for longevity pockets. I knew that in Okinawa, Japan, Drs. Makato Suzuki, Bradley Willcox, and Craig Willcox had already identified a population that produced the longest-lived people in the history of the world. As I quickly discovered, Dr. Gianni Pes, a medical statistician from the University of Sassari, was also tracking down centenarians on the island of Sardinia in Italy. In the island's mountainous interior, which he referred to as the "blue zone," he found a cluster of villages that produced about 10 times more centenarians per capita than the United States. (I liked the term "blue zone" and evolved it to denote any confirmed longevity hot spot around the world.) Later, Dr. Michel Poulain confirmed Pes's research, and together they published their findings in the journal *Experimental Gerontology*.

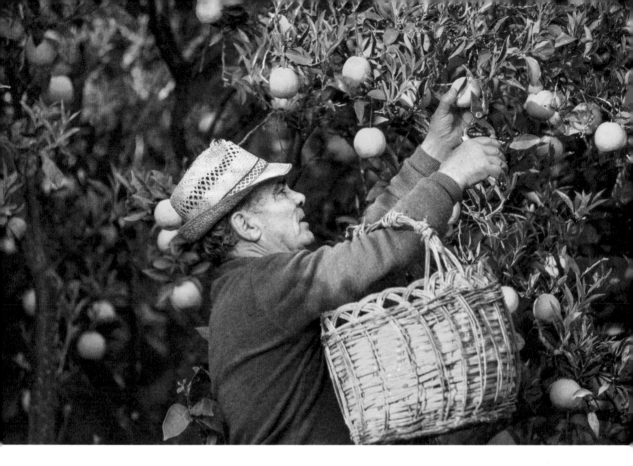

In the United States, Dr. Gary Fraser of Loma Linda University was publishing findings from the Adventist Health Study, research that followed more than 30,000 Seventh-day Adventists in Loma Linda, California, for some 20 years. He found that adherents of the church were living about seven years longer than their Californian counterparts.

Later, with grants from the National Geographic Society, I led projects to discover longevity hot spots on the Greek island of Ikaria and on the Nicoya Peninsula of Costa Rica. In a 2005 cover story for *National Geographic* and in my 2008 book *The Blue Zones: Lessons for Living Longer From the People Who've Lived the Longest,* I profiled each blue zone and distilled the common denominators: The residents of these hot spots were mostly eating a whole-food, plant-based diet, and instead of trotting off to the gym, they moved naturally every 20 minutes or so. Daily rituals like prayer, ancestor veneration, and napping also helped them downshift and lower stress-induced inflammation. And long before people were talking about the social determinants of health, I attributed Sardinians' longevity to their propensity for keeping their aging parents nearby—extending life expectancy for both grandparents and grandchildren—

Many older residents of Sardinia's blue zone keep active by tending small orchards on their properties.

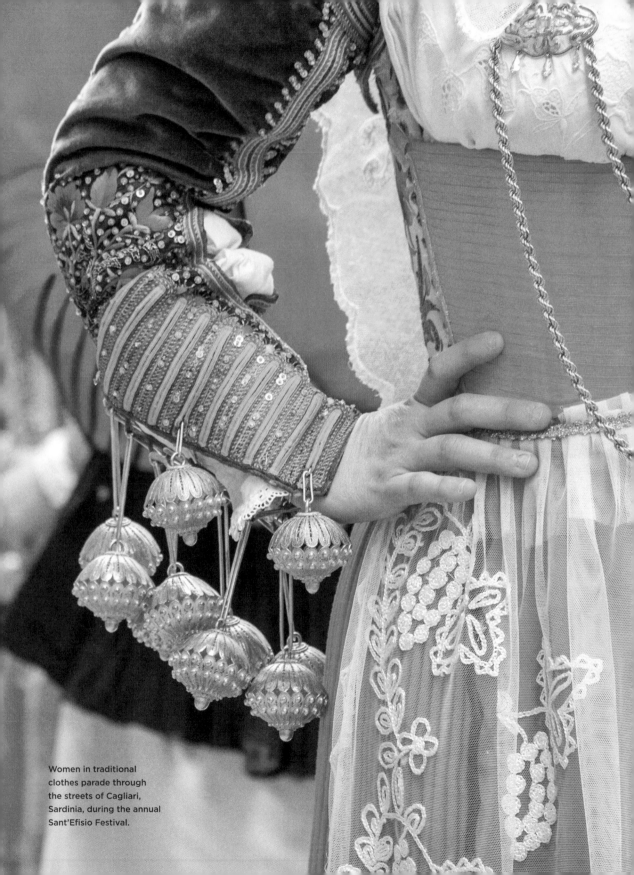

Women in traditional clothes parade through the streets of Cagliari, Sardinia, during the annual Sant'Efisio Festival.

and Okinawans' to their social support groups (called *moais*) and their sense of purpose *(ikigai)*. (See chapter 7 for more on the determinants of longevity.)

The Blue Zones brand of longevity didn't promise that it could help you outlive the biological limits of the human machine. Fact is, the current maximum life expectancy for people in developed nations (i.e., those not beleaguered by infectious diseases such as malaria, dysentery, and cholera) is about 93 years—less for men and a little longer for women. But in the United States, life expectancy is only 77. We are leaving 16 years on the table. "Why?" I wondered.

The answer wasn't that people in blue zones had better genes or superior bodies. Most of them didn't. Rather, they avoided the chronic diseases that foreshorten our lives here in America, from diabetes to cardiovascular disease to dementia to certain types of cancers. They avoided these diseases not because they possessed more discipline or a greater sense of individual responsibility, but rather because

> **THEY DIDN'T PURSUE HEALTH AND LONGEVITY AS IF IT WERE A CHORE. *THEIR HEALTH AND LONGEVITY STEMMED FROM THEIR SURROUNDINGS.***

they lived in environments that made it easier for them to do so. In other words, they didn't pursue health and longevity as if it were a chore. *Their health and longevity stemmed from their surroundings.*

This insight changed everything. It meant that if we wanted to help improve the health and longevity of Americans, we needed to focus on the environments in which they lived—their communities, workplaces, and homes and the businesses they patronized—rather than trying to change their behaviors.

I started to think about applying what I'd learned in blue zones to make life better here in the United States—to "manufacture" a blue zone of our own. Decades ago, the National Institutes of Health funded a half dozen "heart healthy" projects in cities throughout the country, where communities tried to implement diets, exercise programs, and health education. In each case, the researchers saw small improvement in heart health indicators in the short run, but all the efforts failed to show improvement in the long run.

I decided to try a different approach. My goal wouldn't be to change people's behavior, but rather to shape their environments to make healthy choices the easiest ones. In 2008, with a grant from AARP, I put together a team to give it a try. We chose Albert Lea, Minnesota, a community of 18,000 people. The mayor, city manager, school superintendent, local hospital, and business leaders all pledged their support for the project.

With some of the most talented experts in the country, we developed a policy bundle to improve the walkability and bikeability of Albert Lea and slowly transform the city's street designs from car-friendly to people-friendly. We put together a school program that favored healthy foods over junk foods. We persuaded restaurants and grocery stores to make healthy foods easier to find and more enticing to eat. We introduced a Blue Zones Pledge for individuals that eventually enrolled 25 percent of the city's adult population into volunteering and taking workshops on how to pursue their sense of purpose. Finally, we developed a process to help like-minded people get together in walking groups—not only to get them out moving but mostly to build new friendships. We knew that if we could organize friends around healthy behaviors, those behaviors were more likely to stick.

The first Blue Zones Project ran for about 18 months. "The results were remarkable," Harvard's Dr. Walter Willett told *Newsweek* magazine. As data gathered by Gallup showed, we raised the life expectancy of the average citizen by three years and shaved about 30 percent off the city's year-over-year healthcare bill. The project worked not because we tried to change 18,000 people's minds. We changed their surroundings.

Since then, we've brought the Blue Zones Project model to 72 cities across the country, from Fort Worth, Texas, to Naples, Florida, as well as to the entire

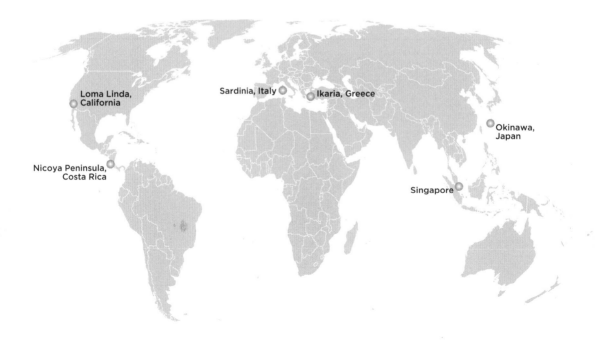

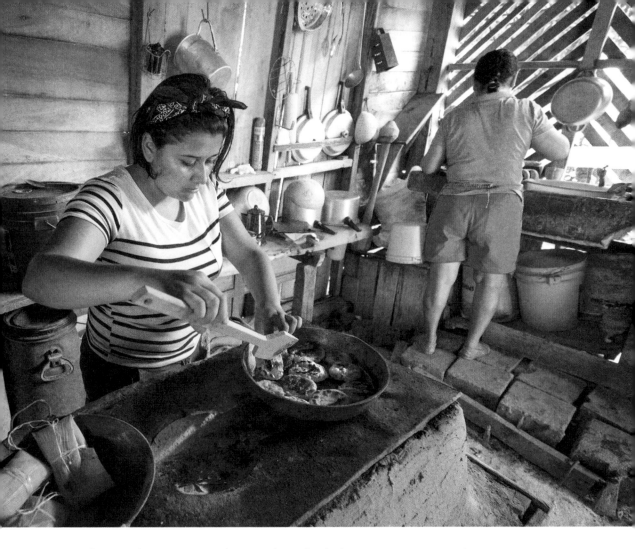

states of Iowa and Hawaii. We're changing things for the better—one community at a time.

———————————

Nearly 20 years after I first landed in Sardinia with a backpack and a *National Geographic* assignment, I returned to all the blue zones to produce a four-part series for Netflix. Like everywhere else in the world, the blue zones have changed—mostly because of modernization and the devastating impact of American food culture. But a bevy of scientists continue to study them. Dr. Luis Rosero-Bixby has been tracking the health of the residents in the Nicoya Peninsula. Fraser continues to mine the decades-long Adventist Health Studies for new dietary guidelines. Suzuki and the Willcoxes continue to monitor Okinawa's centenarians. Pes, who I believe is the world's greatest longevity expert, is still at work in the mountain villages of Sardinia, where

Relatives of a centenarian prepare a meal in his home on the Nicoya Peninsula of Costa Rica.

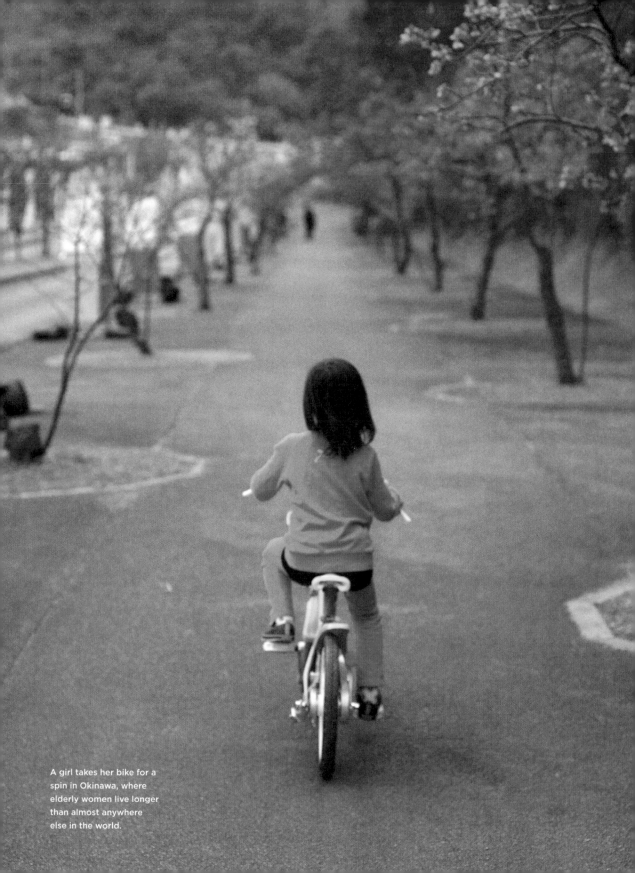

A girl takes her bike for a spin in Okinawa, where elderly women live longer than almost anywhere else in the world.

strong traditions and remote locations continue to preserve the factors that make them extraordinary. And in Ikaria, Romain Legrand, a researcher from Dijon University Hospital, published a survey of people over age 85 that confirms the importance of socializing, taking naps, swimming, gardening, and more.

We added a new blue zone to our coverage, too. During my visits to Singapore for a *National Geographic* story on happiness, I marveled at the tiny country's success in proactively improving the quality of life of its citizens. Indeed, when I examined their health statistics, I found that since 1965 their life expectancy had increased by an astounding 35 years. Singaporeans now enjoy the world's longest disease-free life expectancy.

Despite traveling with a production crew of some 20 people for the Netflix series, I occasionally had time during my journeys to reflect on my many experiences in the blue zones. I recalled nostalgically the 30-some trips I've taken over the years, the experts who've helped me along the way, and the many centenarians I've met—almost all of whom are gone now. I wrote almost 100 pages of notes during the four months of filming and in the process realized that I had gleaned more insights about the blue zones. Those notes have inspired this book.

> I RECALLED NOSTALGICALLY THE 30-SOME TRIPS I'VE TAKEN OVER THE YEARS, THE EXPERTS WHO'VE HELPED ME ALONG THE WAY, AND THE MANY CENTENARIANS I'VE MET.

Late one night in Singapore, jet-lagged and wired-tired, I wrote the following in my journal: *Though we in the United States live in the most prosperous country in the history of the world, we're more overweight, divided, and unhealthy than ever. Life expectancy has dropped every year for the past four years, as has overall happiness. So, if more prosperity doesn't seem to be working for us, what else could?*

My thoughts returned to the blue zones, where I'd learned the priceless value of slowing down, of engaging in long conversations with a neighbor, of unrushed family dinners, of eating low off the food chain, and of cooking at home. I recalled the counterintuitive joy of getting out from behind my steering wheel and back onto my feet. Of walking to the places I need to go—and if they were too far away, of moving closer to them. Of gardening instead of weight training. Of getting closer to family, to beauty, to nature, and to the rhythms of life that have set the tempo for the human species for the past 25,000 generations.

I hope this book inspires you to find something equally rewarding in your own life.

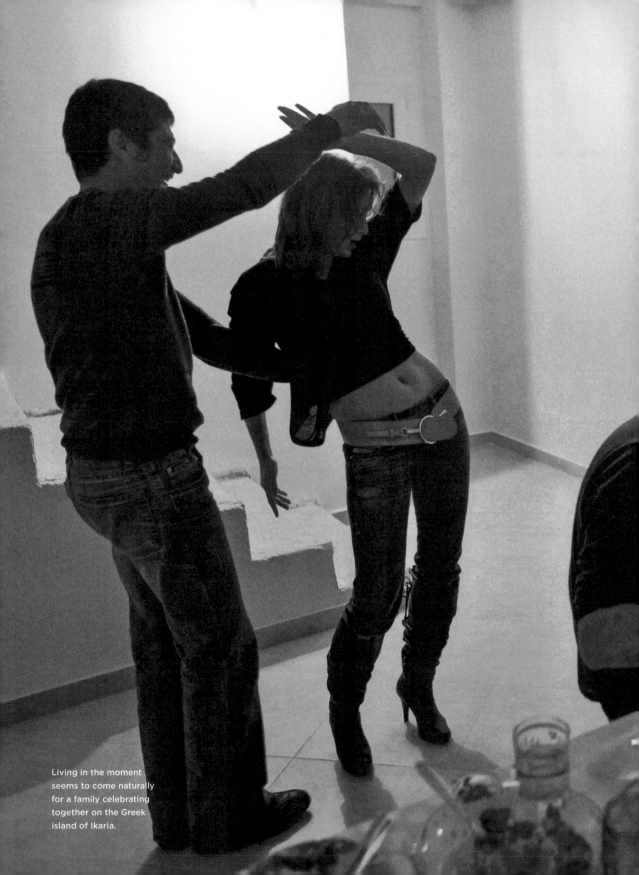

Living in the moment seems to come naturally for a family celebrating together on the Greek island of Ikaria.

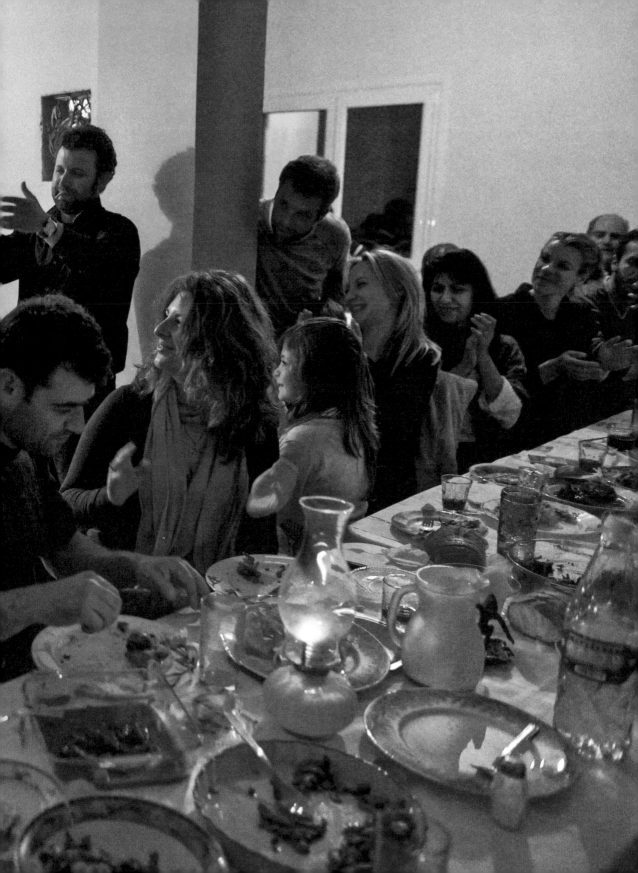

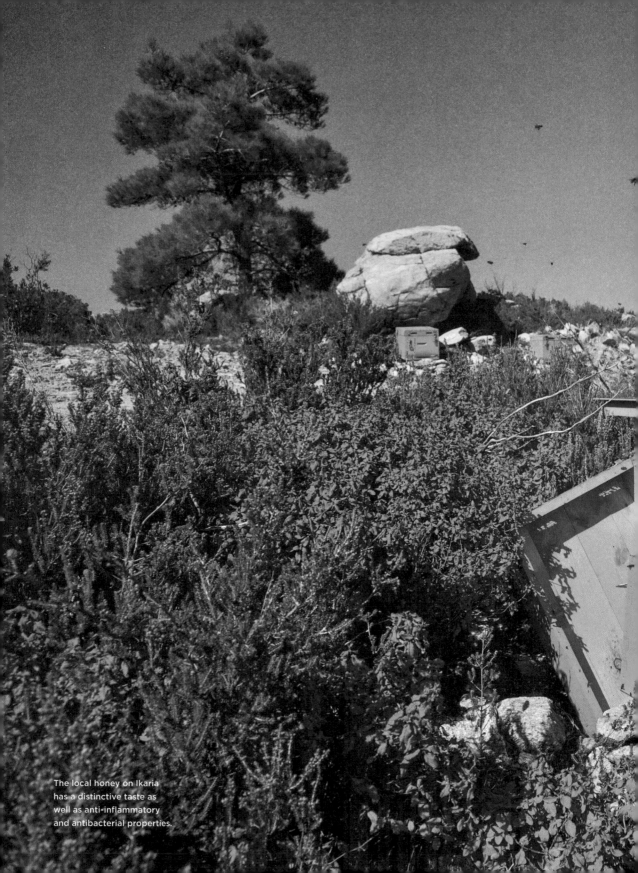

The local honey on Ikaria has a distinctive taste as well as anti-inflammatory and antibacterial properties.

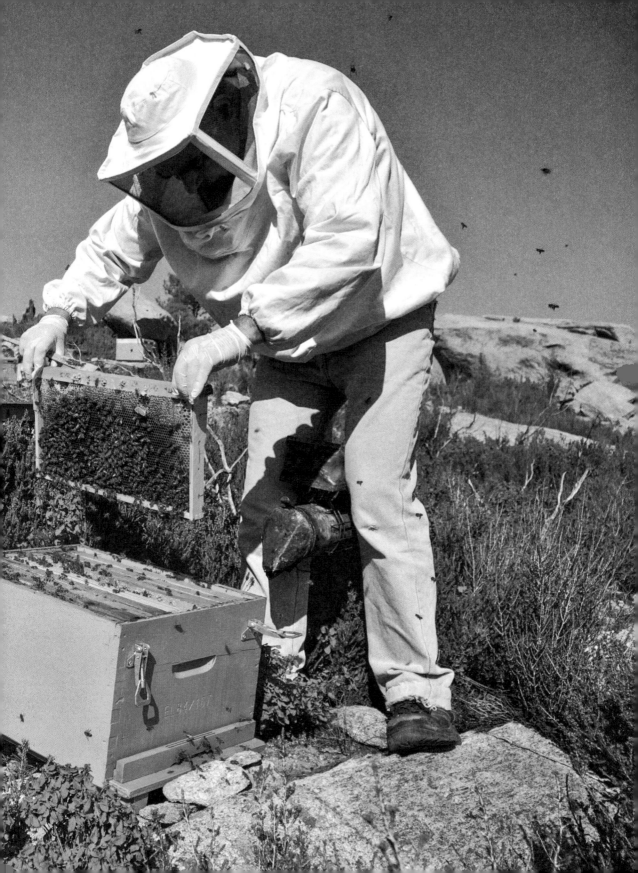

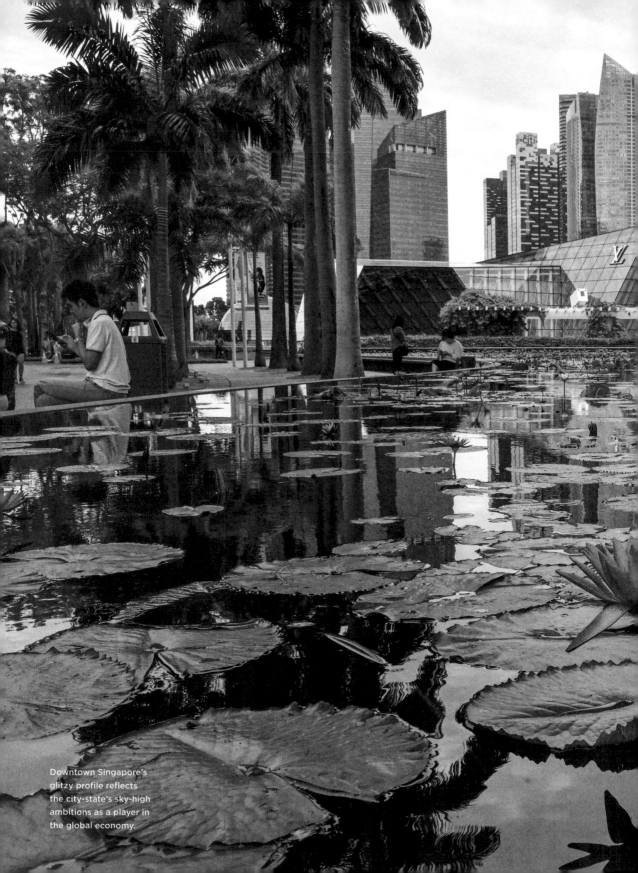

Downtown Singapore's glitzy profile reflects the city-state's sky-high ambitions as a player in the global economy.

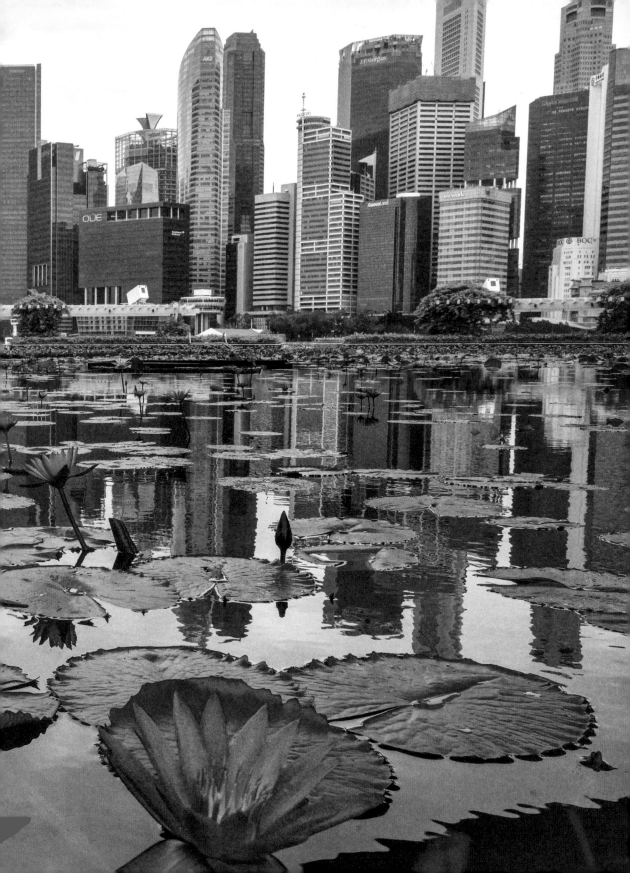

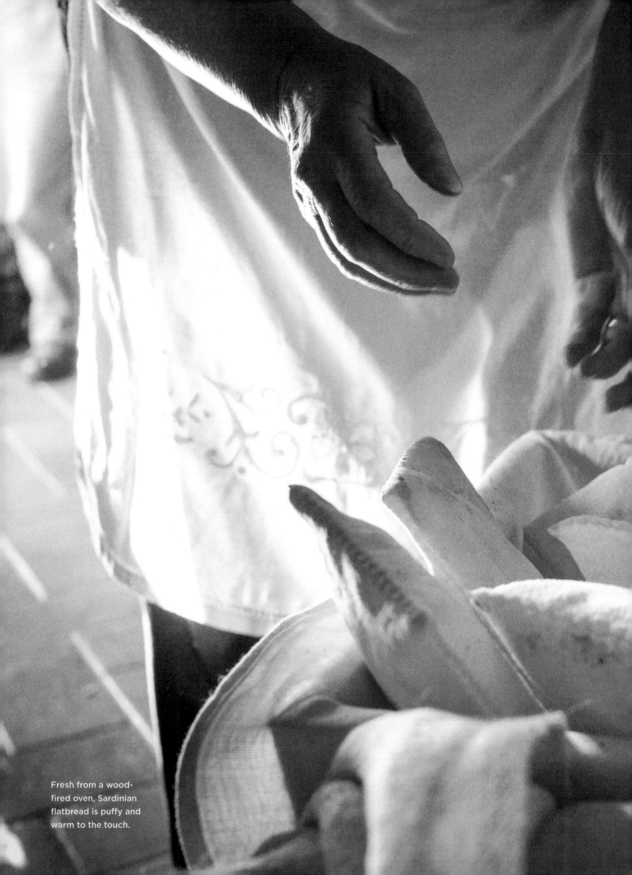

Fresh from a wood-fired oven, Sardinian flatbread is puffy and warm to the touch.

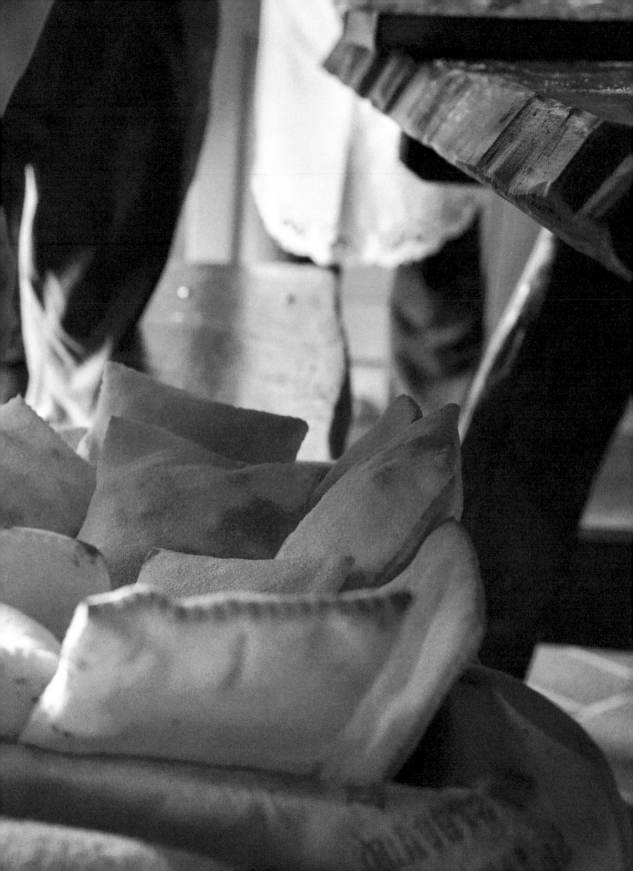

# PART I

# The Blue Zones

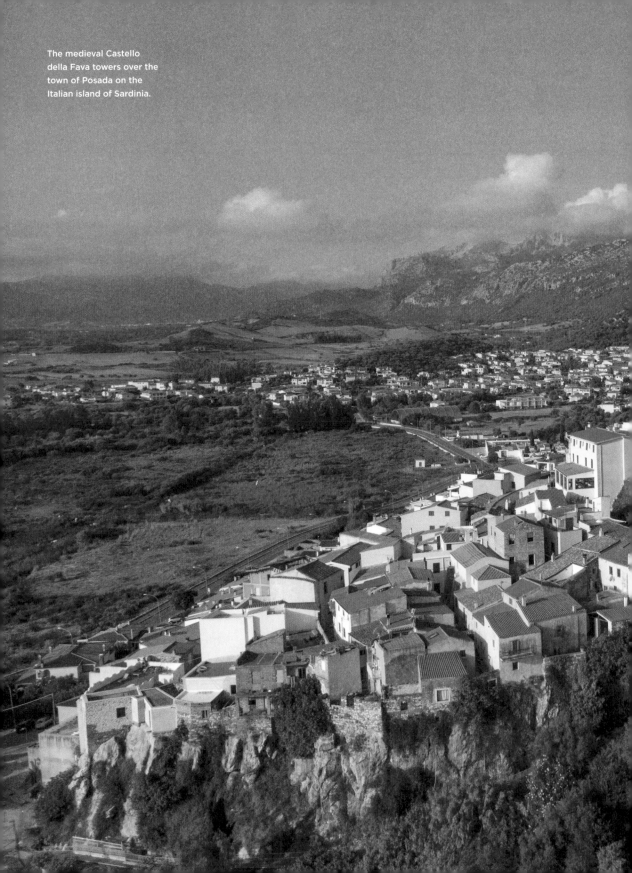

The medieval Castello della Fava towers over the town of Posada on the Italian island of Sardinia.

CHAPTER 1

# Sardinia

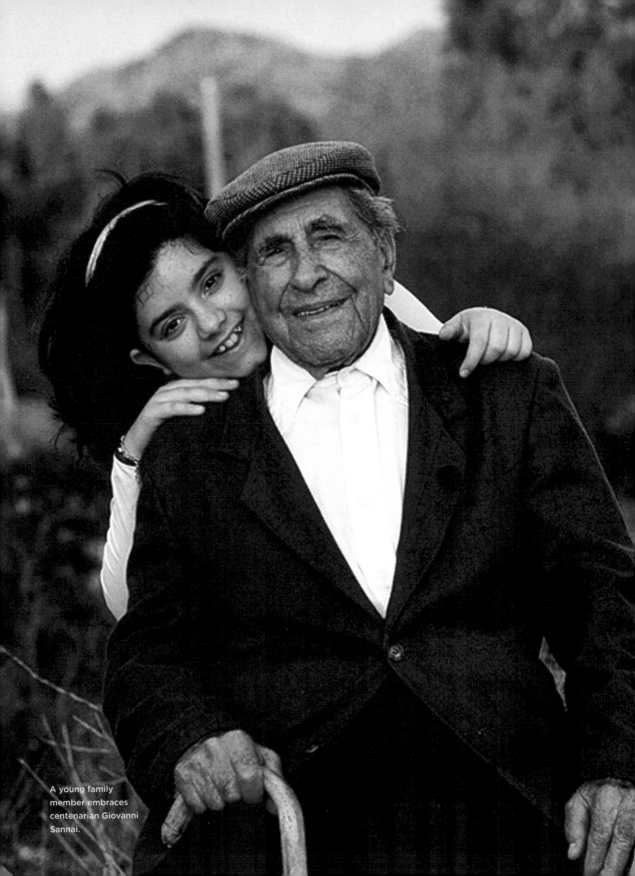

A young family member embraces centenarian Giovanni Sannai.

# Island of Long Life

From the air, the mountain town of Villagrande Strisaili looks like a burnt-orange splash on a vast carpet of green. Up close, its whitewashed houses, bars, and bakeries cascade down steep cobblestone streets. With only 3,200 people, Villagrande is the largest of six villages in the Sardinian blue zone, a kidney-shaped region at the center of the island that the world has long recognized as a hot spot of longevity. Of the 17,865 people born between 1880 and 1900 in these six villages—which include Arzana, Baunei, Seulo, Talana, and Urzulei as well as Villagrande—at least 91 have lived to see their 100th birthday, a rate that exceeds what you'd expect to find in the United States by a factor of 10.

Here in the blue zone, centenarians are treated like local heroes, their portraits painted on murals lining the streets. Everybody knows who they are and cheers them on. When I returned to the town recently with my friend Gianni Pes, a medical statistician from the University of Sassari, we found a banner strung across the front of the house we were visiting. It proclaimed, *"Buon 101° Compleanno Zia Giulia*—Happy 101st Birthday Aunt Giulia." Inside we found Giulia Pisanu seated at a round table with five loving nieces and a nephew. She wore a blue sweater over a floral blouse and a big smile on her face.

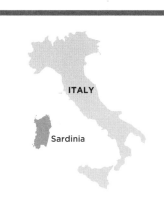

- The island's blue zone is concentrated in a cluster of mountain villages.

- The rate of centenarians produced in Sardinia is 10 times that in the United States.

- The traditional diet of Sardinia's shepherds was mostly bread and cheese.

- The genetics of Sardinians may favor longevity.

"I'm never lonely," she said, gesturing at her family.

"She's almost like a mother to us," said Teresa Pisanu, the oldest of the nieces, who were all in their sixties and seventies.

For years now, Giulia's nieces have rallied around their super-aging aunt. Every day at least one of them helps her with chores around the house or comes by just to keep her company. As I glanced around the sitting room, I noticed a single bed tucked against the wall. That's where the nieces sleep when it's their turn to stay with Aunt Giulia, they explained.

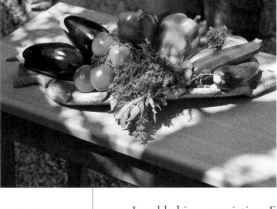

Locally harvested vegetables and herbs are key components of the Sardinian diet.

"What we're doing is nothing special," said Teresa. "We make sure she eats well, we help her bathe, and we get her out to spend time with friends and family."

"You probably get something out of it, too," I ventured.

"We don't think of it that way," she said. "It's not even a question for us. We do it because that's what family does."

I nodded in appreciation. Ever since my first visit here 20 years ago, I'd been struck by the fierce loyalty Sardinians demonstrate toward their families, especially toward their elders. As I noted in my 2008 book, *The Blue Zones,* you won't find any long-term care facilities in these communities. They don't warehouse their seniors in nursing homes as we often do in America. Here, respect increases with age. Younger generations feel an affectionate debt to their parents and grandparents. In fact, of the 50 or so centenarians I interviewed decades ago, all but one had a daughter or granddaughter actively caring for them.

In a place like Villagrande, elders living with their families are expected to pitch in with childcare, cooking, gardening, or some other activity that contributes to the functioning of the household. This gives them a strong sense of purpose and self-esteem. Far from being put out to pasture by their families, they are loved—and love in return.

"This is so important," said Pes, who has interviewed more than 500 centenarians here and around the world. "Her family keeps her engaged mentally and socially."

Along with the Belgian demographer Michel Poulain and Luisa Salaris of the University of Cagliari, Pes was the first researcher to prove that male centenarians in Villagrande excelled as the world's longest-lived men. In most parts of the globe, female centenarians outnumber their male counterparts by more than four to one. In Villagrande, the ratio is almost one to one.

Plus, as Pes pointed out, the elderly in Villagrande tend to stay mentally sharp until the end. Only 19 percent of people here over the age of 90 suffer any form of dementia, compared with 33 percent in the United States. "The lesson of this blue zone is that dementia is not necessarily an inevitable event for the elderly," he said.

So, what's their secret?

To tease out the factors responsible for Sardinia's extraordinary longevity, Pes has conducted extensive lifestyle surveys with centenarians and their families throughout the island since the 1990s. From a mountain of data about his subjects' medical histories, diet, physical activities, and family lineage, he'd zeroed in on a few likely suspects.

One was lucky genes. As his surveys showed, many centenarians also had

Sweet and savory potato tarts emerge hot from the oven.

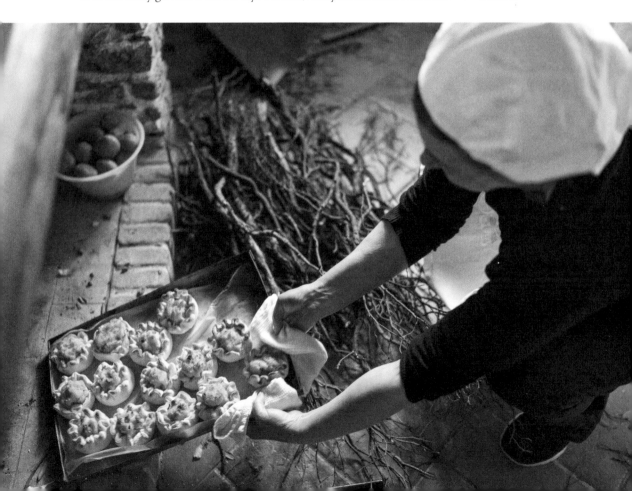

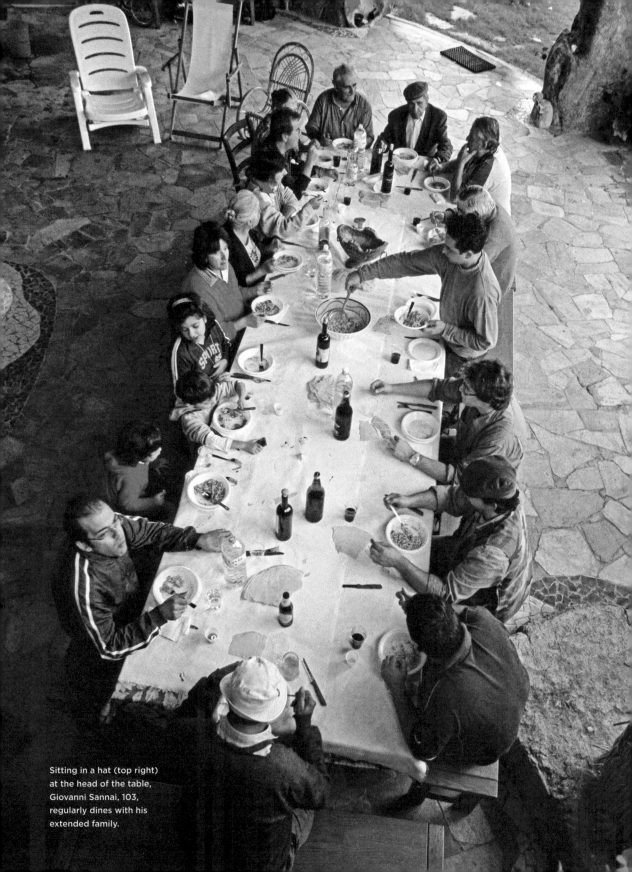

Sitting in a hat (top right) at the head of the table, Giovanni Sannai, 103, regularly dines with his extended family.

a long-lived brother, sister, or parent, suggesting a possible genetic influence. Previous studies had revealed that the people of Sardinia were genetically distinct from those in the rest of Europe. Could the region's self-imposed isolation have created a genetic incubator of sorts, amplifying some traits and subduing others to create a formula for longevity?

The original Sardinians came from Iberia, according to Paolo Francalacci, an evolutionary anthropologist from Sassari University who has studied the DNA of the islanders. About 14,000 years ago, a small band of genetically related people migrated to Sardinia with a distinct genetic marker, the M26 lineage of the Y chromosome. "This genetic marker is found in 35 percent of the Sardinians today and is very rare elsewhere," he said.

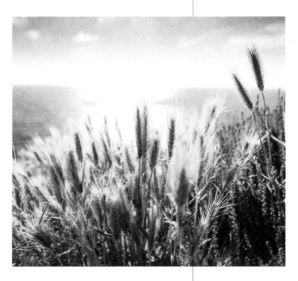

Cereal grains like barley grow wild on the rugged slopes of Sardinia.

A few of the traits Sardinians inherited from these ancestors were negative, such as a higher incidence of type I diabetes and multiple sclerosis. But others were positive, like resistance to malaria and higher longevity rates. Put genetic isolation together with cultural isolation, and you get some very interesting results, Francalacci said: "The people there maintained not only their genetic features, but also their economic isolation and traditional social values, such as the respect for elders as a source of experience, the importance of the family clan, and the presence of unwritten laws—all of which proved to be effective means for avoiding foreign domination over the centuries."

Could this particular environment have interacted with Sardinia's unique set of genes to create a population of super-aging men?

Maybe. But Pes had his doubts. Too many other findings failed to support the genetic explanation. "Consider, for instance, the genes of inflammation," he said. "We expected to find something interesting in Sardinian DNA. We studied several tens of gene variants related to inflammation, but we didn't find any evidence of their role in the survival of Sardinians. The same for genes related to cancer and those related to cardiovascular disease."

Not only that, but the spouses of Sardinian centenarians also lived longer than the siblings of centenarians, he found. This suggests that the diet and

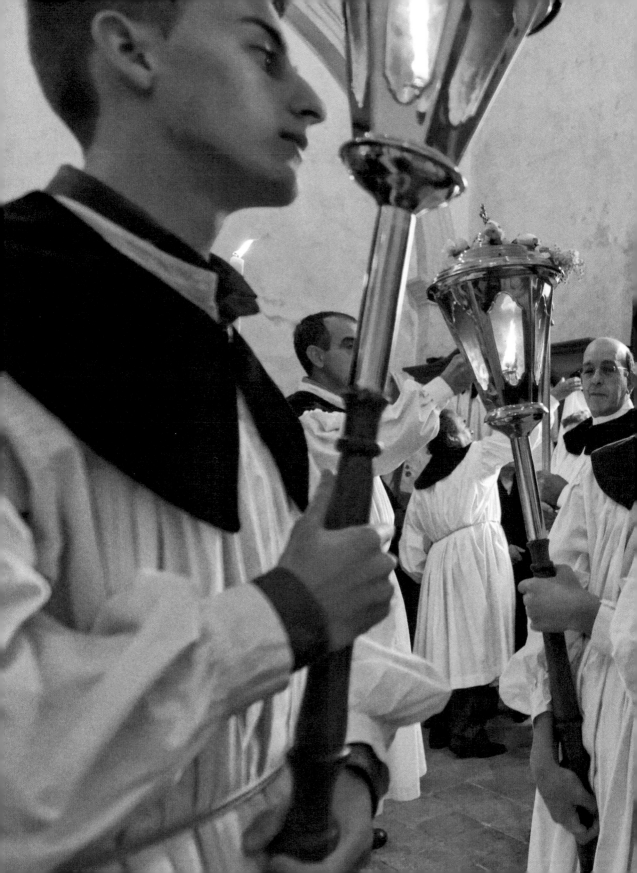

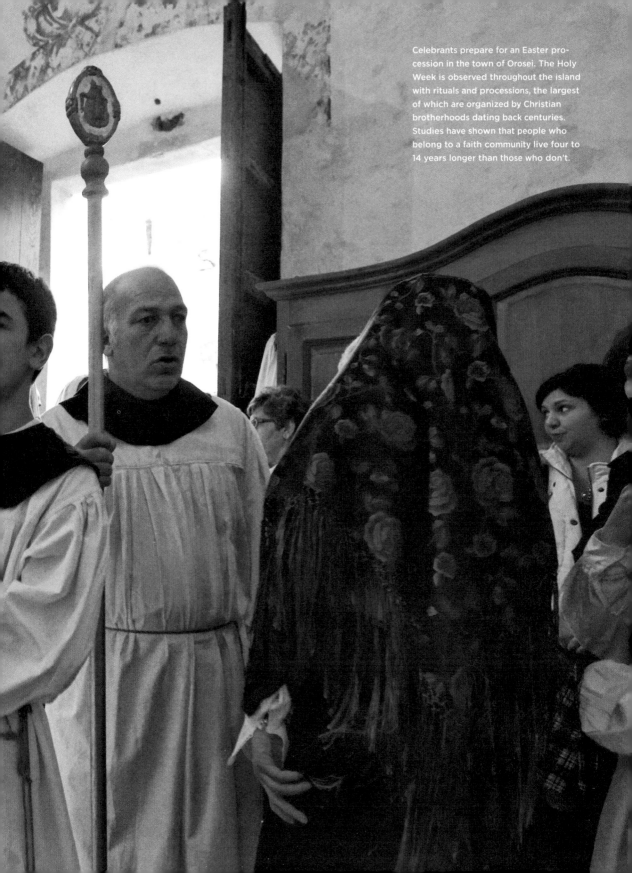

Celebrants prepare for an Easter procession in the town of Orosei. The Holy Week is observed throughout the island with rituals and processions, the largest of which are organized by Christian brotherhoods dating back centuries. Studies have shown that people who belong to a faith community live four to 14 years longer than those who don't.

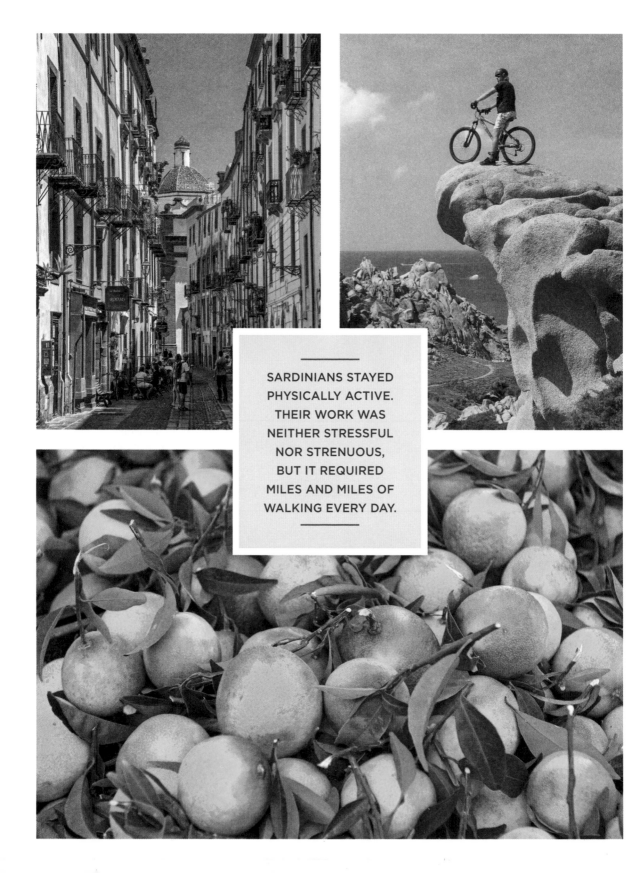

SARDINIANS STAYED
PHYSICALLY ACTIVE.
THEIR WORK WAS
NEITHER STRESSFUL
NOR STRENUOUS,
BUT IT REQUIRED
MILES AND MILES OF
WALKING EVERY DAY.

lifestyles shared by couples might have had a greater influence than genetics on health and long life.

Focusing on the diets of centenarians, Pes combed through dozens of nutrition surveys from the early 20th century. These surveys, conducted by public health personnel, revealed that back in the day, Sardinians ate an extraordinarily simple diet. One survey from 1941 reported that people mostly consumed bread. "Peasants leave early in the morning to the fields with a kilogram of bread in their saddlebag ... At noon their meal consists only of bread, with some cheese among wealthier families, while the majority of the workers are satisfied with an onion, a little fennel, or a bunch of ravanelli [radishes]. At dinner, the reunited family eats a single meal consisting of a vegetable soup [minestrone] to which the richest add some pasta."

Below: Villagers celebrate the annual Festival of the Redeemer in the mountain town of Fonni.

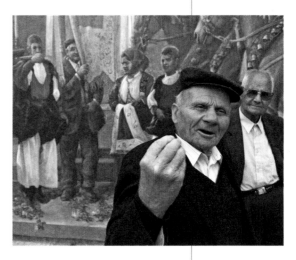

This practice changed after World War II when soldiers returned from mainland Italy with a taste for the Mediterranean diet, including pasta, more fruits and vegetables, and moderate amounts of meat, mostly pork and lamb. Pes speculated that this dietary shift may have provided blue zones villagers with a much needed bump in nutrients at just the right time in their lives to achieve their remarkable life spans.

Since then, unfortunately, American influences have flooded the island with chips, sodas, sugary yogurts, pizza, and burgers, nudging out fruits and fresh vegetables. Even Villagrande now has its own share of pizza joints and ice-cream parlors. A predictable rise in the rates of obesity, diabetes, and heart disease has followed.

All the same, when analyzing blood samples from Sardinians who still adhered to a traditional diet, Pes found a few potential new clues to their successful aging. "Something interesting is happening in the guts of the elderly," he said.

In the Sardinian blue zone, people over age 90 have twice as much of a special type of fatty acid in their blood as other Italians. This substance, called odd-chain saturated fatty acid, has been associated with lower risks of cardiovascular disease, diabetes, and chronic inflammation, among other conditions.

Opposite (clockwise from top left): Quaint villages, rocky views of the ocean, and fresh produce count among the many charms of Sardinia.

But it doesn't come from the consumption of cheese, milk, or any other ingredient in the traditional Sardinian diet. More likely, Pes speculated, it's being synthesized by the microbiota in their gut, possibly during the fermentation of fiber. If true, that would represent yet another benefit of consuming mainly plant-based foods.

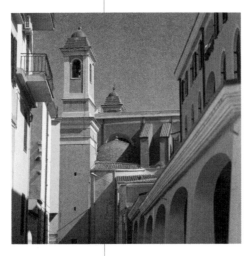

Researchers have also found a greater diversity of bacteria in the gut of centenarians than you'd expect, Pes added. Generally, as we age, the number of species diminishes, given changes in diet, lifestyle, and the use of antibiotics. But in Sardinia, an analysis of microbiota from elderly residents revealed an even greater diversity than normal—more like what you'd find in the gut of a 60-year-old. Yet another sign of delayed aging in the blue zone.

By contrast, the level of thyroid hormones in the blood of Sardinian centenarians was unusually low, Pes said. Although these hormones are essential to human growth and metabolism, reduced thyroid function has also been associated with increased longevity. One theory is that this deficiency is due to a lack of iodine. As Pes pointed out, photos of Sardinian women from a century ago show the prevalence of goiters (an enlarged thyroid), which are caused by an iodine deficiency. But another explanation points to the Sardinian diet, which includes significant amounts of cruciferous vegetables, such as cauliflower, broccoli, cabbage, and kale. Although the connection has yet to be proved, these types of foods contain compounds suspected of affecting thyroid function.

The food habits of Sardinians aren't the whole story when it came to their

**Towers overlook Castello, the old-town quarter of Sardinia's capital, Cagliari.**

## SARDINIAN FLATBREAD

One of the most distinctive Sardinian foods, *pane carasau*, is a crisp, thin bread that is shaped in rounds. Owing to its appearance and crackling sound, it is also called "sheet music" bread *(carta de musica)* in other parts of Italy. This bread dates back to ancient times, when shepherds herding their flocks needed a food that would not go bad while they were away from home for long stretches. In Sardinia, pane carasau graces the table at almost every meal and forms the base of many other dishes. Traditionally, village women make the bread once a month in a group effort.

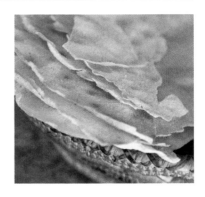

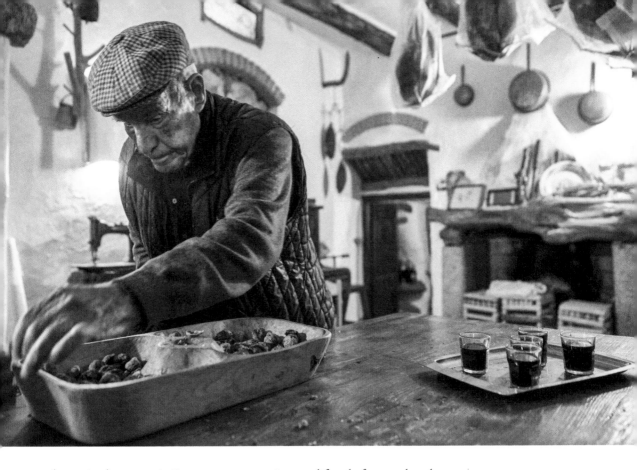

longevity, however. As Pes was eager to point out, lifestyle factors also play a significant role, including the occupations of the longest-lived men. An analysis of his questionnaires revealed two factors closely associated with longevity.

The first was that Sardinians stayed physically active. Fifty years ago, most of the men in the blue zone were either shepherds or farmers who spent their days in constant motion. Their work was neither stressful nor strenuous, but it required miles and miles of walking every day. This low-intensity exercise may help explain why these shepherds turned out to be 10 times more likely to live to 100 than men in the rest of Italy.

The second was the steepness of the blue zone environment. To move their animals from the highlands to the plains, the shepherds had to hike up and down the rocky Gennargentu Mountains. Back home in their villages, every trip to a store, to a bar, or to visit friends meant more climbing up and down steep streets.

There is a lesson here for the rest of us, Pes suggested. We tend to think that the path to good health requires intense, adrenaline-infused workouts. But when we overwork our muscles, we flood our cells with free radicals that

In the Ogliastra region of the island, a man prepares food and wine while waiting for a group of friends.

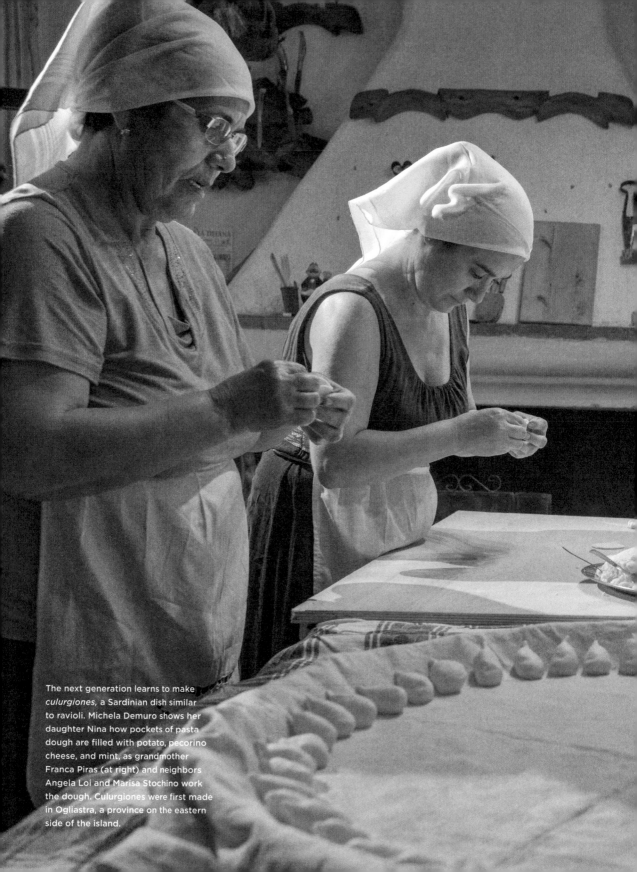

The next generation learns to make *culurgiones*, a Sardinian dish similar to ravioli. Michela Demuro shows her daughter Nina how pockets of pasta dough are filled with potato, pecorino cheese, and mint, as grandmother Franca Piras (at right) and neighbors Angela Loi and Marisa Stochino work the dough. Culurgiones were first made in Ogliastra, a province on the eastern side of the island.

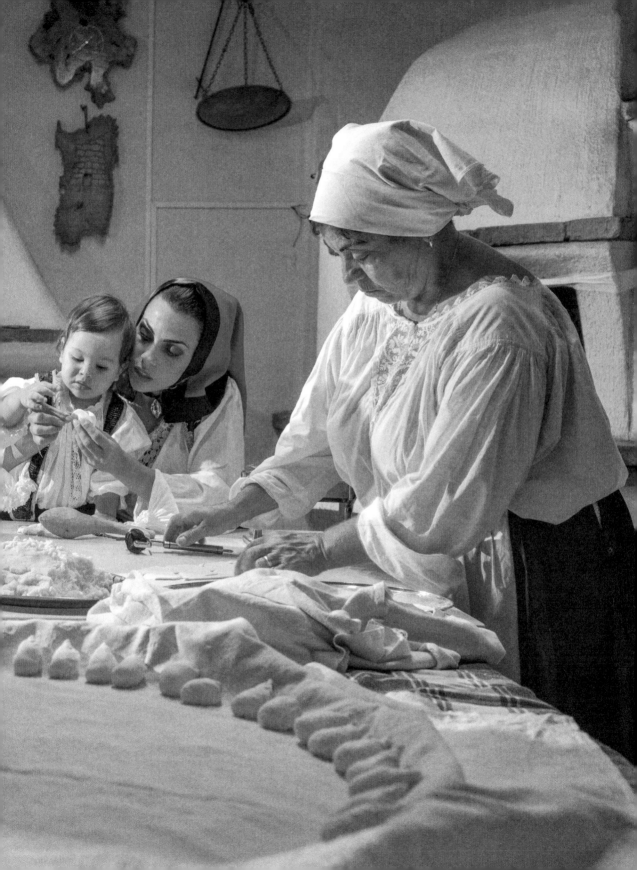

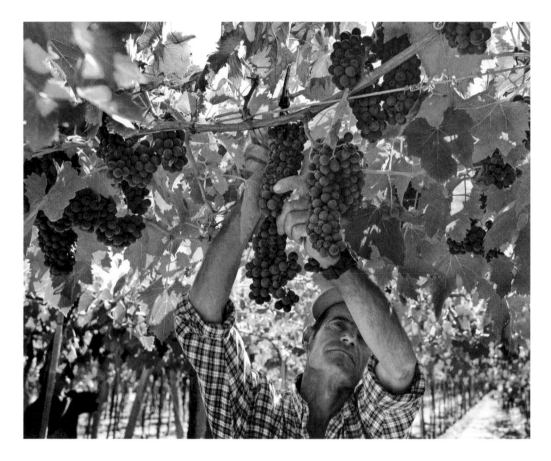

Some of the grapes harvested at Sella & Mosca winery will be used to make Sardinia's distinctive Cannonau wine.

contribute to rapid aging. Sardinian men and women, by contrast, worked their muscles a long time, but they did it in their gardens, with their animals, or by walking back and forth to church. Their lifestyles and environment set them up for success.

Put all these elements together—a unique genetic history, a stubbornly traditional culture, a largely Mediterranean diet, and a lifestyle of constant movement—and you have most of the ingredients necessary for a long, healthy life, Pes said.

But there was one more factor to consider—and it might be the most important.

"It's their attitude," said Pes. "They're optimistic, curious, and conscientious, even to the point of being bossy. It's very rare to find a sad centenarian."

As a study by researchers at the University of Cagliari recently confirmed, centenarians in Sardinia's blue zone rely on frequent social interactions and

# Melis Family Minestrone

TOTAL COOK TIME: 8 HOURS IF USING DRIED BEANS; 30 MINUTES IF USING CANNED BEANS • SERVES 4

Each of the six villages in Sardinia's blue zone prides itself on recipes for both summer and winter minestrones. These fragrant soups not only provide several helpings of vegetables, but they also deliver a full daily dose of beans, my favorite longevity supplement. This bountiful dish is eaten for lunch every day by the world's longest-lived family, the Melises.

In America we tend to eat only the bulbs of fennel, but Sardinians make full use of its aromatic fronds, which are also rich in antioxidants. And, as longevity scientist Gianni Pes points out, a longer cooking time enhances the bioavailability of more nutrients, such as the lycopene in tomatoes, as well as carotenoids and other antioxidants.

7 tablespoons extra-virgin olive oil, divided

1 medium yellow or white onion, chopped (about 1 cup)

2 medium carrots, peeled and chopped (about ⅔ cup)

2 medium celery stalks, chopped (about ½ cup)

2 cloves garlic, minced

One 28-ounce can crushed tomatoes

3 medium yellow potatoes, peeled and diced (about 1½ cups)

1½ cups chopped fennel (bulbs, stalks, and fronds)

¼ cup loosely packed fresh Italian flat-leaf parsley leaves, chopped

2 tablespoons chopped fresh basil leaves

½ cup dried and peeled fava beans, soaked overnight (or one 15-ounce can, drained)

½ cup dried cranberry beans, soaked overnight (or one 15-ounce can, drained)

½ cup dried chickpeas, soaked overnight (or ½ 15-ounce can, drained)

⅔ cup Sardinian fregula, Israeli couscous, or acini di pepe pasta

½ teaspoon salt

½ teaspoon freshly ground black pepper

Warm 3 tablespoons of the olive oil in a large soup pot or Dutch oven set over medium-high heat.

Add the onion, carrots, and celery, and cook, stirring often, until soft but not browned, about 5 minutes. Add the garlic and cook until fragrant, about 20 seconds.

Stir in the tomatoes, potatoes, fennel, parsley, basil, as well as the drained fava and cranberry beans and chickpeas. Add enough water (about 6 to 8 cups) so that everything is submerged by 1 inch.

Raise the heat to high and bring the pot to a full boil. Reduce the heat to low and simmer slowly, uncovered, until the beans are tender, about 1½ hours, adding more water as necessary. If using canned beans, simmer for only 10 minutes.

Stir in the pasta or couscous, salt, and pepper. Add up to 2 cups of water if the soup seems too dry. Continue simmering, uncovered, until the pasta is tender, about 10 minutes.

Pour 1 tablespoon of olive oil into each bowl before serving.

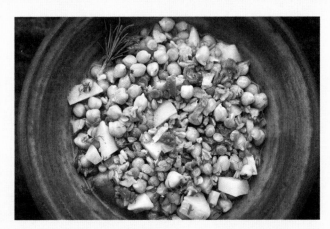

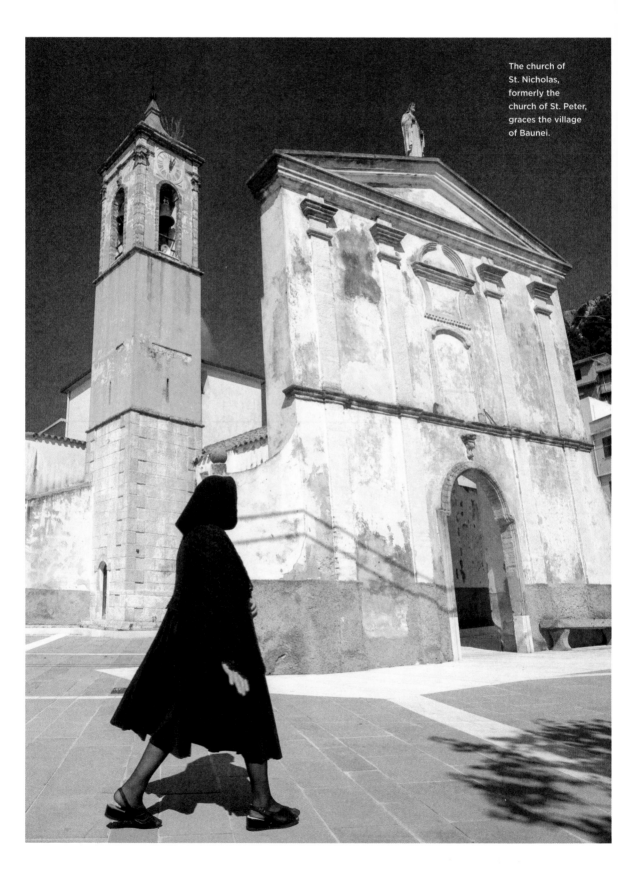

The church of
St. Nicholas,
formerly the
church of St. Peter,
graces the village
of Baunei.

close family bonds to keep their minds sharp and give their lives meaning: "Compared to peers residing in Northern Italy, elderly people from the inner mountainous areas of Sardinia are more physically active, more involved in community social life, have lower loneliness and express greater confidence in their cognitive efficiency, as well as report higher personal satisfaction and emotional competence."

Older people in Sardinia don't retire so much as shift jobs. Men may stop tending sheep, but they'll put their efforts and talents into working in the villages. It's not uncommon to see 90-year-olds on walking patrols or advising city governments. In turn, these expectations that they contribute something to society keep them active and using their brains.

It would be hard to overestimate the importance of family in the blue zone, said Dr. Luca Deiana, who studied centenarians there for more than a decade. Grandparents provide love, child-care, financial help, wisdom, expectations, and motivations to perpetuate traditions and push children to succeed, he said. In fact, all the centenarians I met told me *la famiglia* was the most important thing in their lives—their purpose.

Back at Giulia Pisanu's house, the 101-year-old was showing off the sash she'd been given at her recent birthday party. For her 100th birthday, the town

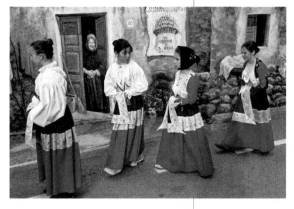

Women and children in the village of Fonni wear traditional dress for the Madonna Dei Martiri Festival.

fathers had presented her with a cake and a commemorative plaque. About five feet two inches tall, and weighing less than 100 pounds, she crossed the room gingerly but with vigor. On her head perched a princess tiara.

"She always tries to make us laugh," said her niece Teresa.

That made Giulia laugh herself, which made her nieces and nephew laugh, too. You could tell that they loved her.

In her role as a local superstar, Giulia has gotten used to speaking with reporters, who always ask her the same question: "What's the secret to long life?"

"Don't be jealous and don't be envious," she told one television correspondent.

That's probably good advice. But to me, the real secret resides in the people surrounding her at the table. You could see it in their beaming faces.

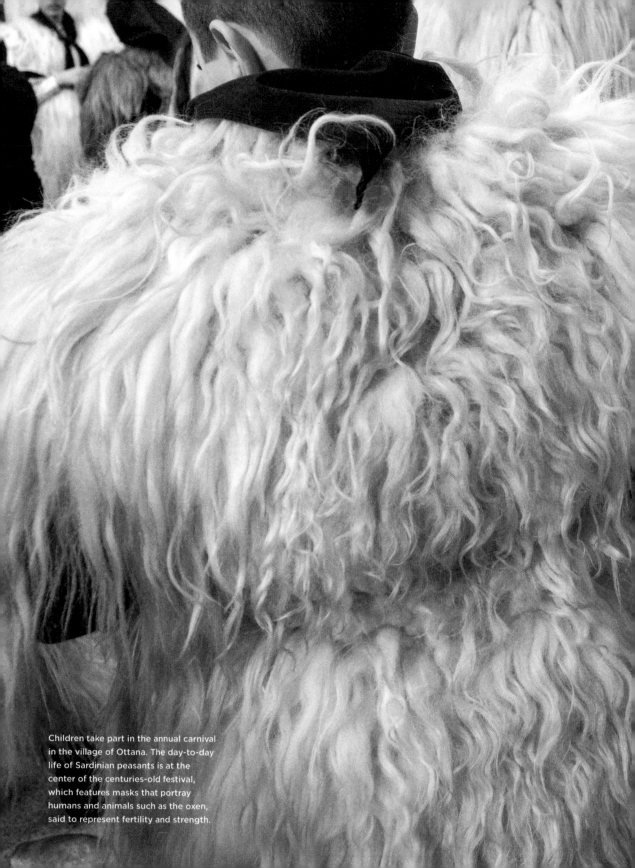

Children take part in the annual carnival in the village of Ottana. The day-to-day life of Sardinian peasants is at the center of the centuries-old festival, which features masks that portray humans and animals such as the oxen, said to represent fertility and strength.

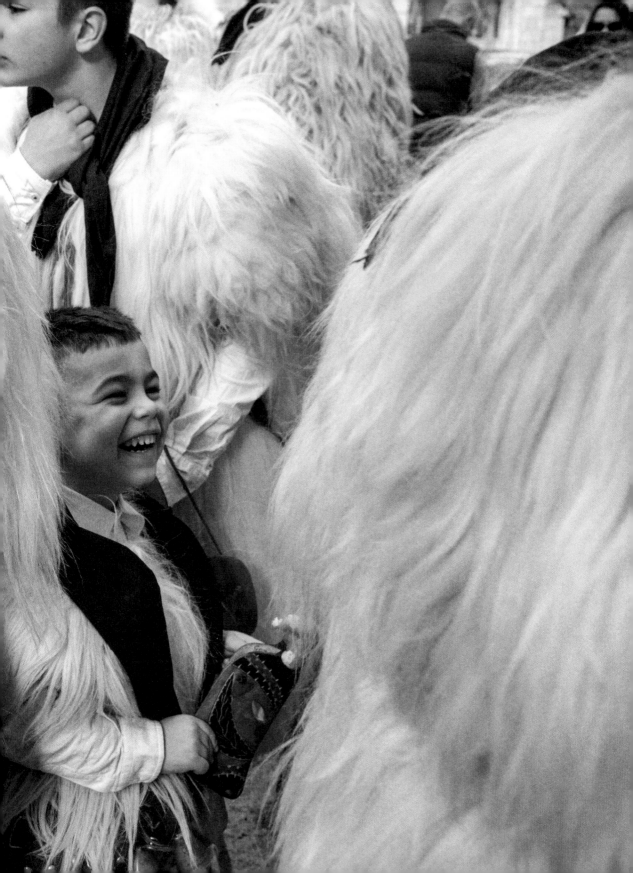

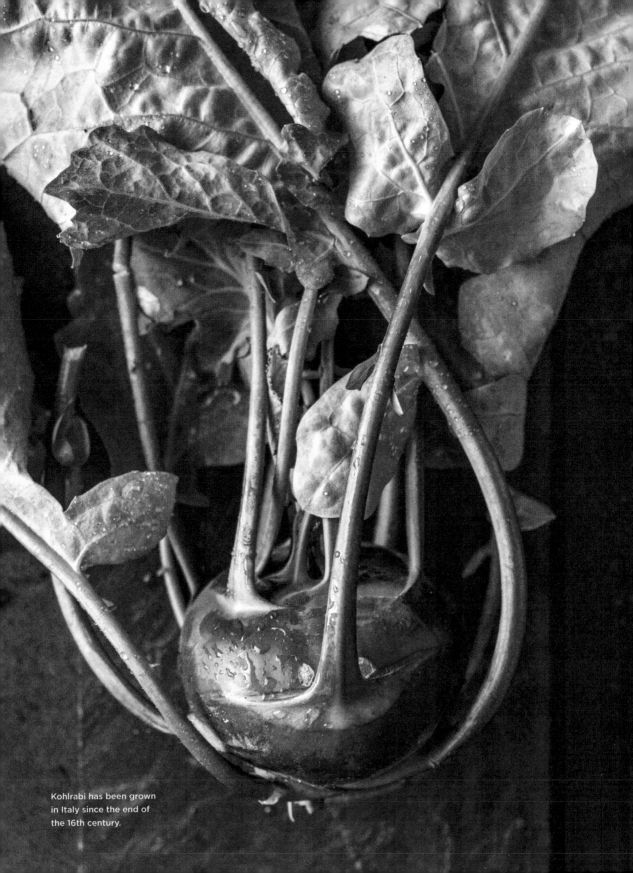

Kohlrabi has been grown in Italy since the end of the 16th century.

# Top Longevity Foods From Sardinia

Although life in the mountain villages of the island's blue zone historically revolved around tending sheep and goats, meat from animals accounted for a relatively small part of Sardinians' traditional diet. Instead, the bulk of their diet consisted of carbohydrate-rich food such as bread, pasta, potatoes, and beans, such as fava beans, supplemented by milk and cheese from goats and vegetables such as tomatoes, onions, zucchini, and cabbage—plus about two small glasses of red wine every day. This low-protein diet began to change after World War II and especially after the 1970s, when American foods like burgers were introduced.

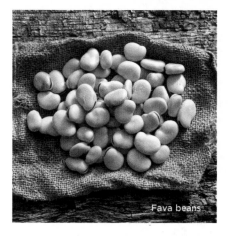
Fava beans

**BARLEY** | Ground into flour for bread or added to soups, barley is the food most highly associated with Sardinian men living to 100.

**FAVA BEANS** | Cooked in soups and stews, fava beans deliver protein and fiber.

**KOHLRABI** | A rich source of fiber and calcium, kohlrabi contains many nutrients, including copper, manganese, iron, and potassium.

**FENNEL** | Rich in fiber and vitamins A, B, and C, fennel is used as a vegetable (its bulb), an herb (its fronds), and a spice (its seeds).

**POTATOES** | Added to minestrone, potatoes help lower cholesterol and reduce the risk of heart disease.

**SOURDOUGH BREAD** | Made from whole wheat and live lactobacillus (rather than yeast), sourdough bread (*moddizzosu*) has a relatively low glycemic index.

**OLIVE OIL** | With healthy monounsaturated fats, olive oil has many longevity benefits, including anti-inflammatory properties.

**ROSEMARY** | Often picked in Sardinian gardens, rosemary helps enhance memory, improve digestion, and prevent brain aging and cancer.

**TOMATOES** | A rich source of vitamin C and potassium, tomatoes are used to make sauces that top Sardinian breads and pasta dishes.

**CANNONAU WINE** | Sardinia's distinctive red wine is made from sun-stressed grenache grapes.

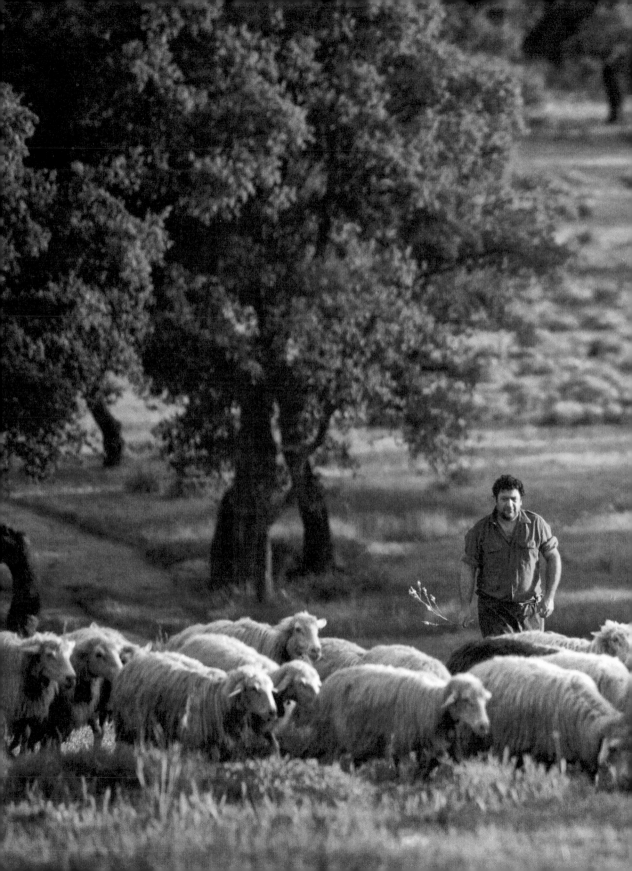

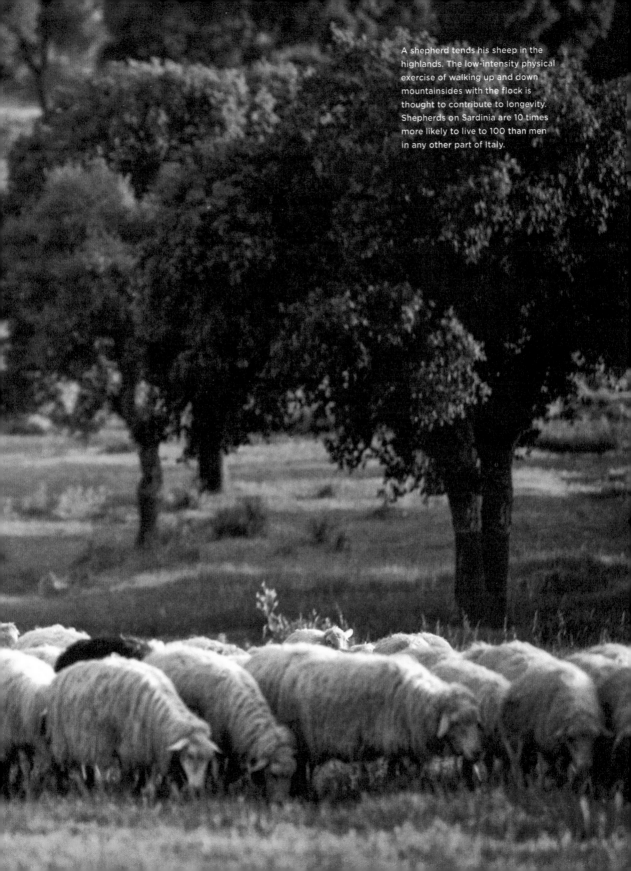

A shepherd tends his sheep in the highlands. The low-intensity physical exercise of walking up and down mountainsides with the flock is thought to contribute to longevity. Shepherds on Sardinia are 10 times more likely to live to 100 than men in any other part of Italy.

# LESSONS FROM SARDINIA'S BLUE ZONE

■ **Eat a "peasant" plant-based diet**

The classic Sardinian diet consists of cheap "peasant foods" like whole-grain sourdough bread, beans, garden vegetables, fruits, and, in some parts of the island, olive oil. Sardinians also traditionally eat pecorino cheese made from grass-fed sheep, whose cheese is high in omega-3 fatty acids. Goat's milk is the dairy of choice, and meat is largely reserved for Sundays and special occasions.

■ **Put family first**

Sardinia's strong family values help assure that every member of the family is cared for. People who live in strong, healthy families suffer lower rates of depression, suicide, and stress.

■ **Celebrate elders**

Grandparents can provide love, childcare, financial help, wisdom, and the expectations and motivation to continue traditions and push children to succeed in their lives. This may all add up to healthier, better-adjusted, and longer-lived children. It may give the overall population a life-expectancy bump.

■ **Take a walk**

Walking five miles or more a day, as Sardinian shepherds do, provides all the cardiovascular benefits you might expect, and also has a positive effect on muscle and bone metabolism without the joint pounding of running marathons or triathlons. If you want to live to 100, you're much better off living in a walkable area than you are running off to the gym three or four times a week. And if you want an extra longevity bump, live in a place where the streets are steep.

■ **Drink a glass or two of red wine daily**

Sardinians drink wine moderately. Cannonau wine has two or three times the level of artery-scrubbing flavonoids as other wines. Moderate wine consumption may help explain the lower levels of stress among men.

■ **Laugh with friends**

Men in this blue zone are famous for their sardonic sense of humor. They gather in the street each afternoon to laugh with and at each other. Laughter reduces stress, which can lower one's risk of cardiovascular disease.

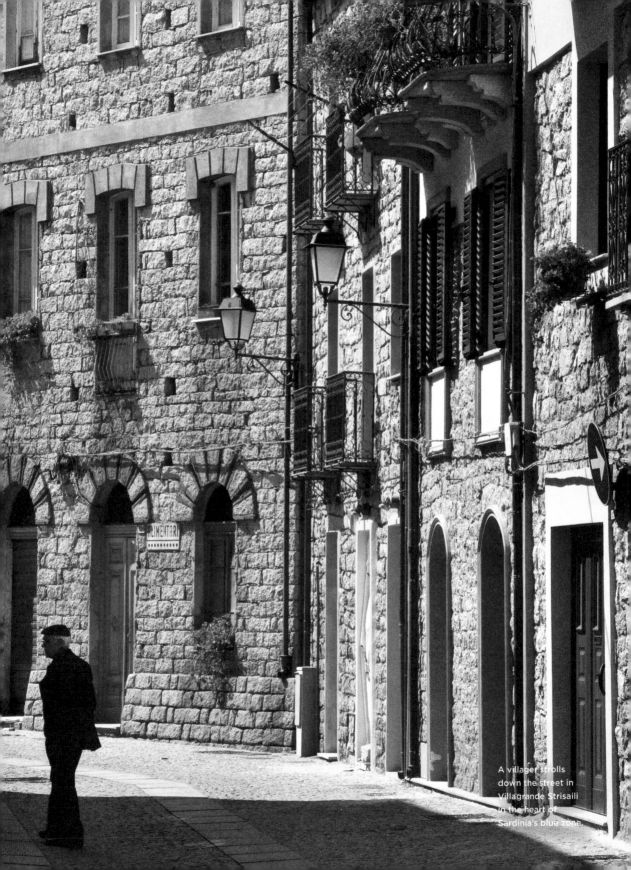

A villager strolls down the street in Villagrande Strisaili in the heart of Sardinia's blue zone.

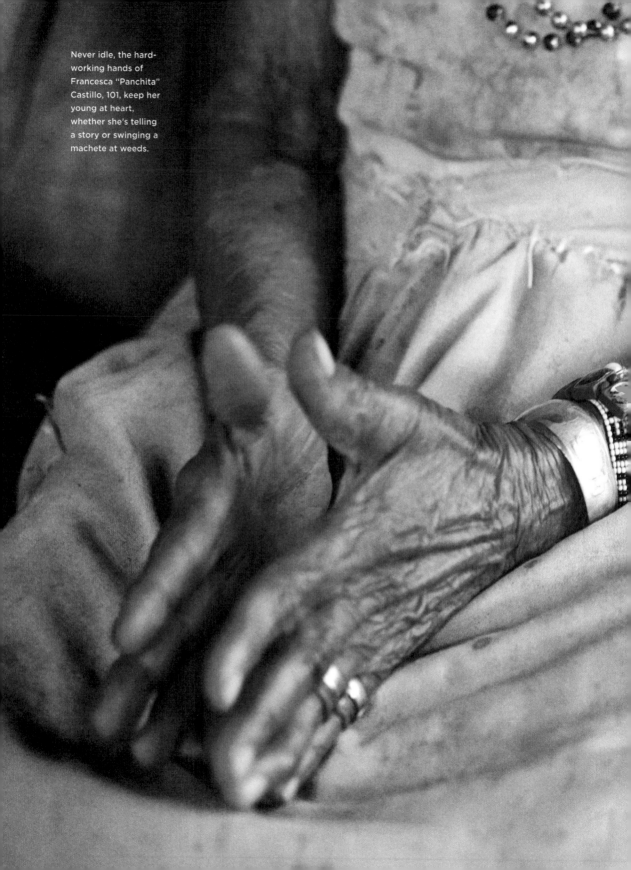

Never idle, the hard-working hands of Francesca "Panchita" Castillo, 101, keep her young at heart, whether she's telling a story or swinging a machete at weeds.

# CHAPTER 2

# Nicoya

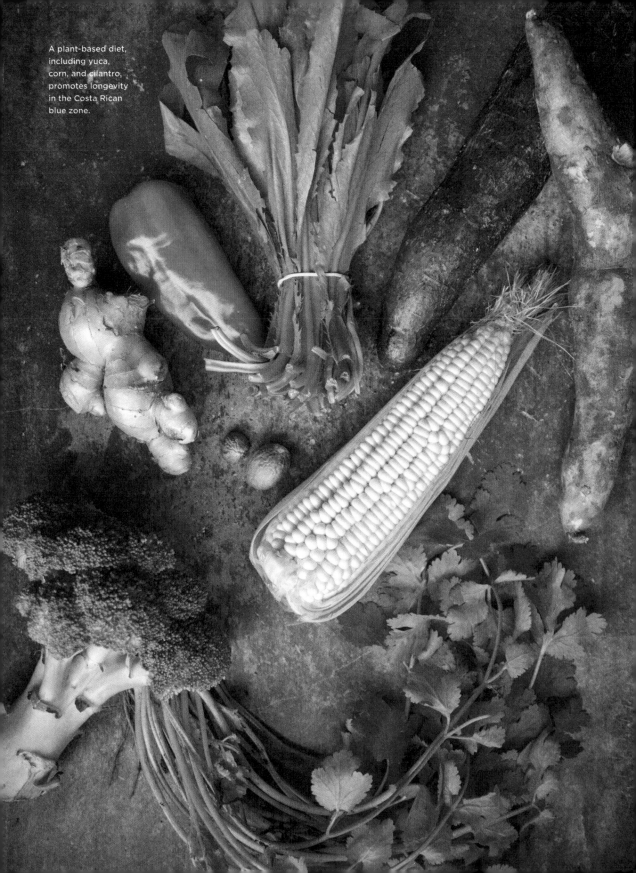

A plant-based diet, including yuca, corn, and cilantro, promotes longevity in the Costa Rican blue zone.

# Costa Rica's Blue Zone

He was resting in a hammock when I arrived. It was a little after nine o'clock in the morning, and José Ramiro Guadamuz had already put in four hours of work. Rising before dawn, he'd downed a cup of black coffee, mounted his horse, and crossed the river to the farm where he pastures his cattle. After milking the cows, he'd watered the herd and returned home for a hearty breakfast of beans and rice with pico de gallo.

That sounded like a busy morning to me when he described it later. But it was just another normal day in the life of this Costa Rican cowboy who turned 100 in August 2022.

Of all the centenarians I've ever met—and I've interviewed more than 300—Don Ramiro struck me as one of the most vital. Dressed in tan jeans and a crisp turquoise shirt and wearing brown-rimmed glasses and a wide-brimmed *sabanero* hat, he rose from the hammock and greeted me clear-eyed and sharp as a tack.

"Funny, I don't feel old," he said, when I remarked on his youthful appearance. "Except for my left arm, of course, from when my horse threw me."

His farmhouse lies at the heart of Costa Rica's blue zone, a 30-mile-long strip along the spine of the Nicoya Peninsula. Mostly dry pastureland and tropical

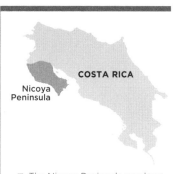

**COSTA RICA**

Nicoya Peninsula

- The Nicoya Peninsula was long isolated from the rest of Costa Rica.

- The region is one of the driest and sunniest in the country.

- Costa Rica's health-care system is among the best in the Americas.

- Nicoyan men are three times more likely to reach age 90 than U.S. men.

forest, the region feels worlds away from the touristy beaches that hug the nearby Pacific coast. Lately, it has attracted global attention because of its reputation as a hot spot of longevity—primarily for men. As researchers have calculated, a Nicoyan man at age 60 has about twice the chance of reaching 90 as a man in the United States, and he has a greater chance of staying healthy even though health expenditures per person in the United States are about 10 times as high as they are in Costa Rica. Women are also long-lived here, though not as dramatically as in other blue zones.

How has this small country, with its limited natural and financial resources, managed to outperform its much larger and wealthier neighbor to the north? That's the question that keeps drawing me and my team of experts back to Nicoya year after year. And what we've discovered here, layer by layer, is a unique blend of genetics, traditional foods, and a robust public health system that—combined with tight family bonds, an active lifestyle, a belief in God, and a sunny dry environment—has helped Nicoyans avoid life-shortening illnesses such as heart disease, cancer, and diabetes better than Americans by a wide margin.

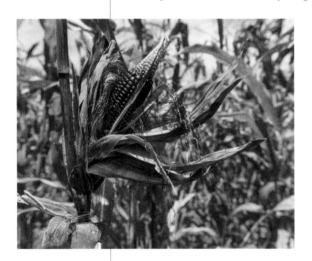

Blue corn, one of the oldest varieties in the Americas, grows on a family farm in Nicoya.

My fascination with Nicoya began in 2006, when Luis Rosero-Bixby, then director of the Central American Population Center in San José, agreed to accompany Michel Poulain and me to the region to investigate its formula for success. The previous July, Rosero-Bixby had given a talk at an international conference in France titled "Costa Rican Nonagenarians: Are They the Longest Living Male Humans?" For his study, he'd systematically combed local birth records and Costa Rica's well-documented death records of the voting population. Meanwhile, Poulain had been studying pockets of other long-lived peoples around the world, including in the mountain villages of Sardinia.

I remember our journey well. Three hours from San José, with Rosero-Bixby at the wheel of a Toyota Land Cruiser, we turned off the Pan-American Highway and drove through ever drier and hotter landscapes. Forests gave way to cow pastures with humped-back Brahman cattle and the massive

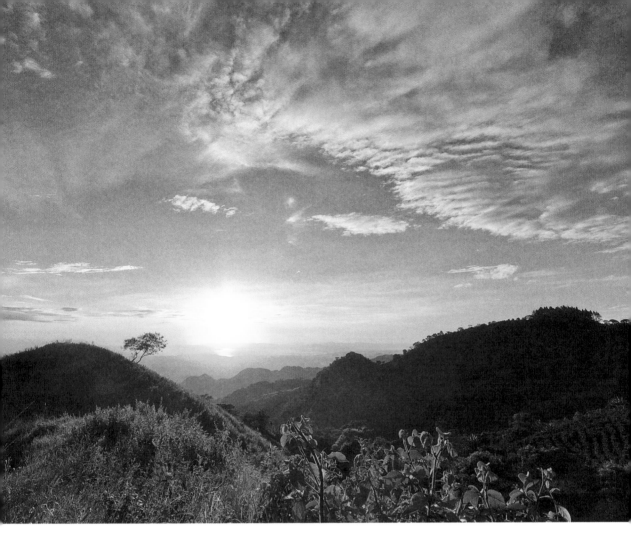

umbrella-shaped guanacaste trees after which the province in the far north-western corner of the country was named.

"Until very recently, this was one of the most isolated parts of Costa Rica," Rosero-Bixby told us as we crossed the bridge over the broad Tempisque River, which separates the Nicoya Peninsula from the mainland. "You can see it's a long way from the highways, and before this bridge was built, most people had to take a ferry to get here."

As was the case in Sardinia, Nicoya's isolation helped preserve its traditional way of life. Until about 50 years ago, most of the men here worked as ranch hands or subsistence farmers, growing their own crops and harvesting tropical fruits, such as sweet lemon, sweet orange (*Citrus sinensis*), and a banana variety called *cuadrado*. For most people, that meant living in extreme poverty, with no electricity or other modern amenities. In fact, Nicoya ranked among

Sunset lights up the tropical forest on the rugged hills facing the Gulf of Nicoya.

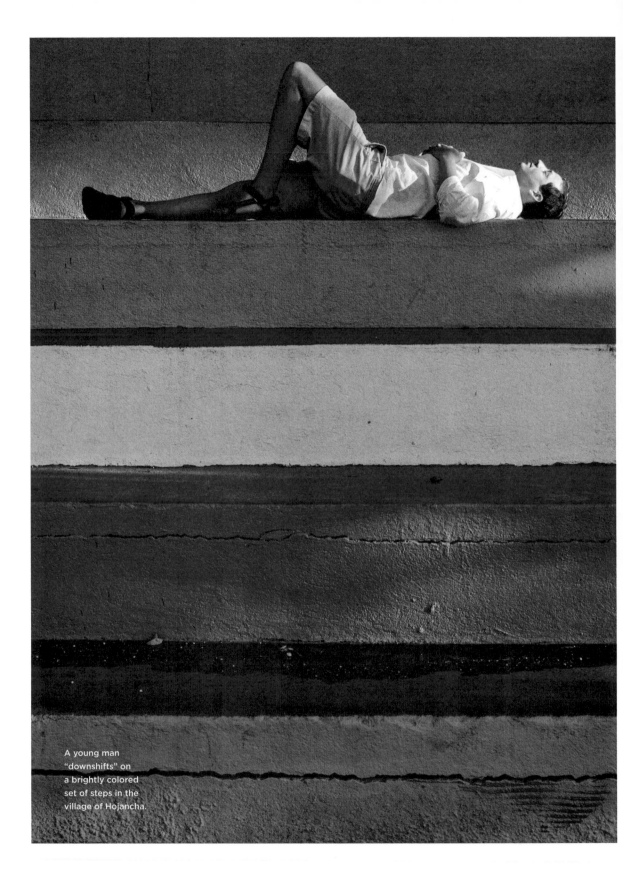

A young man "downshifts" on a brightly colored set of steps in the village of Hojancha.

the poorest regions in Costa Rica, whose per capita income of $12,800 still amounts to only a fourth that in the United States.

Generation after generation, Nicoyans ate what they grew, raised, or hunted. Their low-calorie, low-fat, plant-based diet was largely influenced by that of the Indigenous Chorotega people, who thrived in the region before the Spanish arrived in 1522. The Chorotega lived in simple thatched-hut communities ringed by vegetable gardens, fruit trees, and, farther out, fields of corn and beans. Like other Mesoamerican cultures, they were religious and lived low-stress lives. The cornerstone of their diet was the "three sisters" of traditional Mesoamerican agriculture: beans, corn, and squash. They grew these crops in fields the Spanish called *milpas,* where squash plants provided ground cover to hold in moisture, and bean plants vined up the tall cornstalks.

Although black beans have remained a daily staple in Nicoya, white rice has largely replaced squash in the average diet. Curiously, even though it's lower in fiber and nutrients than brown rice, white rice doesn't cause sugar levels to rise as quickly when eaten with beans. The combination also provides all nine amino acids that our bodies normally need.

Served with corn tortillas and a dash of the Nicoyan hot sauce called *chilero,* beans and rice provide a rich blend of complex carbohydrates, protein, calcium, and niacin. As surveys from the past five decades have revealed, more than two-thirds of the region's traditional diet came from carbohydrates like these—much more than the average American diet today. Only a fifth came from fats, and only a tenth from proteins. Over the course of a day, the average Nicoyan consumes about 1,800 calories, a fourth less than what an American typically consumes.

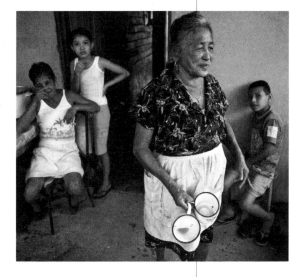

Felipa Muñoz, 86, relaxes at home, where she prepares tortillas before walking five miles to sell them in Hojancha.

Nicoyans may have gotten another nutritional boost from the way they prepared their tortillas. To make the dough called *maíse nixquezado,* they soaked whole corn kernels in calcium hydroxide, or lime and water, which infused the grain with 7.5 times more calcium than normal and unlocked specific amino acids that would otherwise have been unavailable in the corn. As nutritionist Leonardo Mata of the University of Costa Rica explained to me, people who

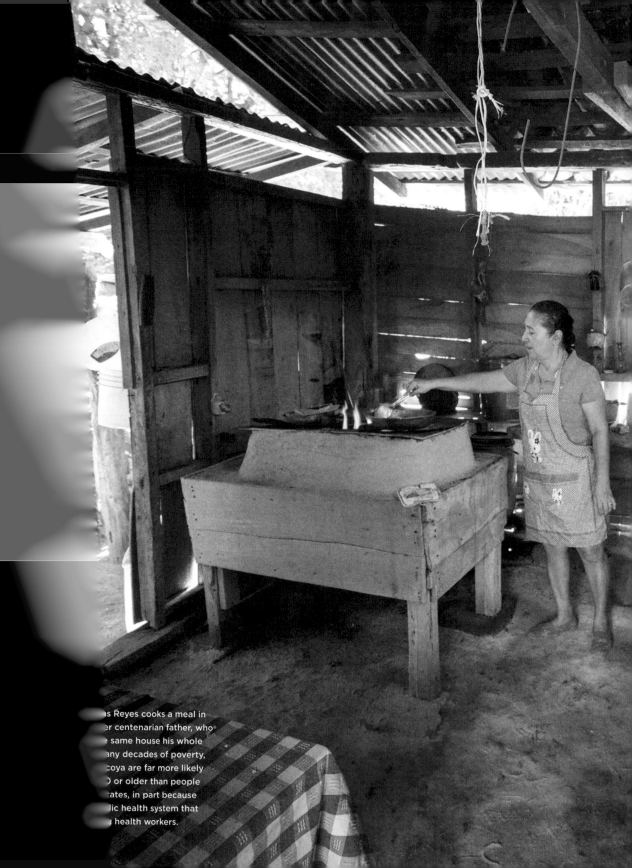

...s Reyes cooks a meal in
...r centenarian father, who
... same house his whole
...any decades of poverty,
...coya are far more likely
...0 or older than people
...ates, in part because
...lic health system that
... health workers.

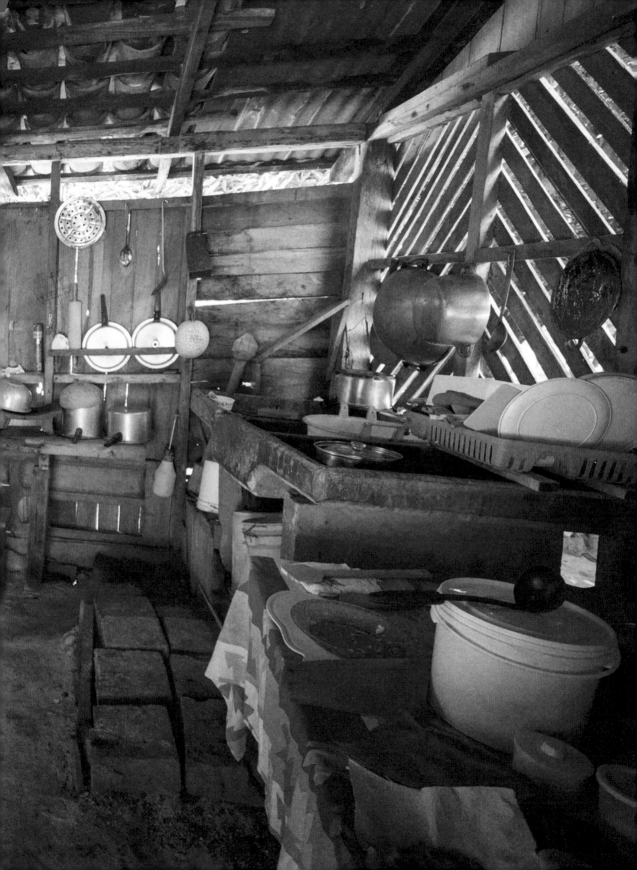

consumed corn prepared this way almost never got rickets and rarely suffered the bone fractures and broken hips that tend to plague older people.

As we met more centenarians in Nicoya, Poulain, Rosero-Bixby, and I identified several other factors at work that might explain their extraordinary longevity. It became clear that the centenarians' deep social networks, their strong faith community, and their habit of regular, low-intensity physical activity also contributed to their success. In addition, they got a healthy dose of vitamin D from sunlight and extra calcium from their water—more, in fact, than from water anywhere else in the country—both of which may have led to stronger bones and fewer falls.

In follow-up studies, Rosero-Bixby looked into how the diet and lifestyle of Nicoyans might have affected their cellular health as well. Together with Stanford University social epidemiologist David Rehkopf and others, he examined blood samples from Nicoya residents aged 60 or older and compared them with samples from other Costa Ricans. They wanted to know if Nicoyan longevity might be explained by differences in their epigenetic profiles.

Epigenetics refers to molecular processes that affect how your genes work. Behaviors like smoking, diet, and stress can change these processes, which are known to affect your health and aging. These changes accumulate over your lifetime, making them reliable markers of your biological age, as opposed to your age in years.

The researchers discovered that Costa Ricans as a whole were almost seven years younger epigenetically than they were chronologically. Centenarians were almost 13 years younger. When compared with other Costa Ricans, Nicoyans also had unique epigenetic patterns in their cells, with fewer types of changes than their fellow citizens, the researchers found.

In a related study, Rehkopf turned his attention to the protective caps, called telomeres, on the ends of Nicoyans' chromosomes. Telomeres wear down over time, which means they can be used as rough markers of biological age. As Rehkopf told me, the telomeres of Nicoyans showed they were up to a decade younger biologically than their chronological age.

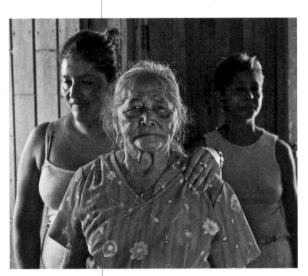

Below: Felipa Muñoz enjoys a moment with her daughter and granddaughter. The love and support of family is key to longevity.

Opposite (clockwise from top): A green bundle of culantro, an herb related to cilantro, adds a strong flavor to Nicoyan stews. At a produce market, José Alberto Guevara Pérez leans over a bin of yuca and purple sweet potatoes. Breadfruit is a plant-based substitute for fish in a delicious poke bowl.

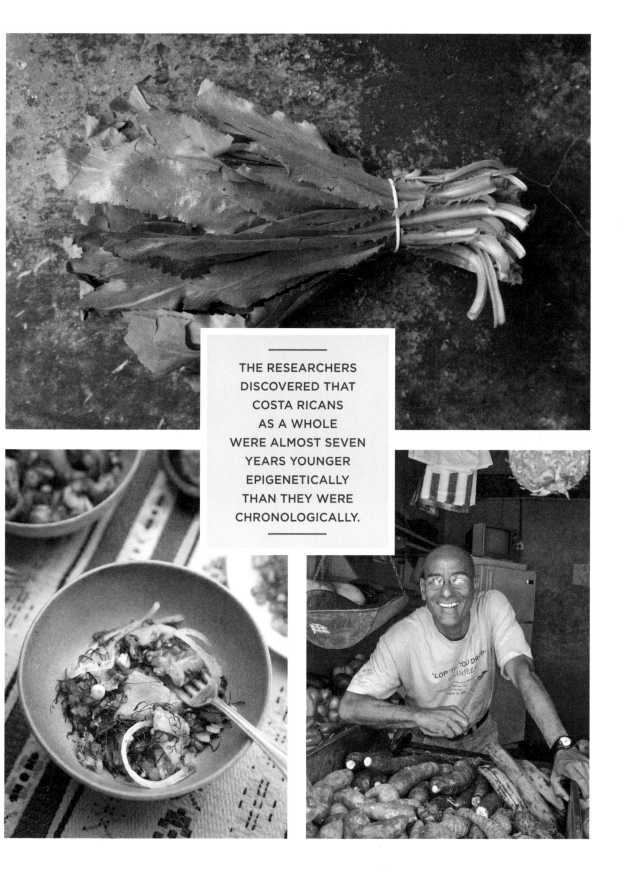

THE RESEARCHERS
DISCOVERED THAT
COSTA RICANS
AS A WHOLE
WERE ALMOST SEVEN
YEARS YOUNGER
EPIGENETICALLY
THAN THEY WERE
CHRONOLOGICALLY.

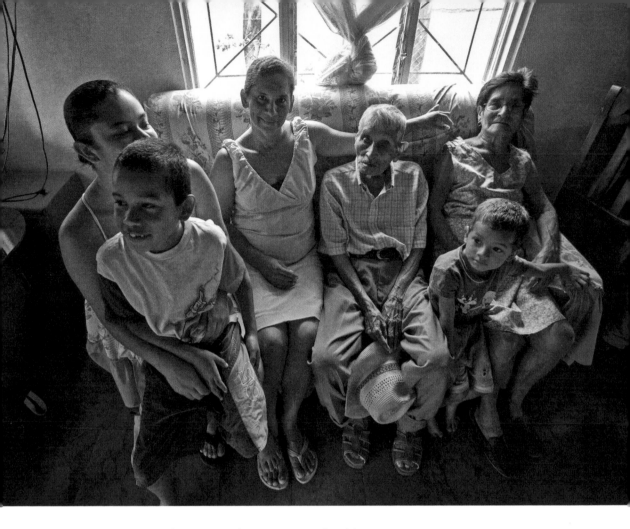

Five generations of family surround Faustino Dinarte Vallejos, 103, on a couch in his home.

So, what was causing this delay in aging?

"A lot of factors affect our aging clocks, not one thing," said Rehkopf, after he joined me in Costa Rica recently. "Diet has been shown to influence our epigenetics, especially fiber and a plant-forward diet. Stress and social connections also have an impact. I remember having conversations with people here in Nicoya about them being happy with what they had and rolling with adversity."

More recently, Rosero-Bixby and his colleagues have found new evidence that consumption of traditional Nicoyan foods—especially grains such as rice—may help explain the region's extraordinary longevity. Significantly, they determined that the population with the longest telomeres in Costa Rica was also that with the lowest household income. As I mentioned earlier, poverty has long been a fact of life in Nicoya, which might help explain why the DNA of the region's elderly has stayed younger than their years.

It might also be possible that Nicoyans' extra years of healthy life are a happy side effect of their strong social and family ties. As we know, belonging to a family relieves stress and gives you purpose and a positive outlook—what Costa Ricans call *plan de vida*. Rosero-Bixby and his colleagues discovered that Nicoyans in general were less likely than other Costa Ricans to live alone. Among those who did, their telomere advantage went *poof.*

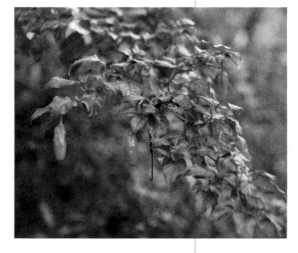

By this measure, Venerando López was a wealthy man. His daughters and their families lived just down the hill from him and his wife, Rosa, in a dusty compound off a mountain road south of the town of Nicoya. Although they had no electricity or refrigeration—he and Rosa kept their food in a basket dangling from the ceiling to protect it from rodents—

Nicoyans often grow sweet red peppers in their backyards.

they had each other and their family. Most afternoons, once his work was done, Venerando would get a visit from one of his daughters or a grandchild or two. Otherwise, he'd sit on his porch, listen to the birds, and thank God for being alive at 99.

"I'd like to live a little more, because this world is so beautiful," he said when we joined him on the porch late one morning while Rosa was down with the grandkids. Venerando wore a pale button-down short-sleeve shirt, gray pants, and a gray porkpie hat. When he laughed, which was often, he revealed his few remaining teeth.

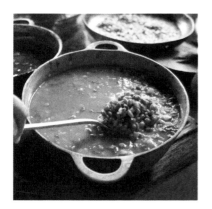

## THE THREE SISTERS: BEANS, CORN, SQUASH

Nicoya's plant-based diet—which tends to be low in calories, low in fat—was strongly influenced by the Chorotega people, who lived in the region before the arrival of the Spanish in the early 16th century. Like other Mesoamerican cultures, the Chorotega thrived on the "three sisters" of traditional agriculture: beans, corn, and squash. Squash provided ground cover for the bean plants, whose vines climbed the corn stalks. In return, bean plants also fixed nitrogen in the soil to help fertilize the corn. Although Nicoyans today have largely substituted white rice for more traditional squash in their meals, they still enjoy black beans as a daily staple.

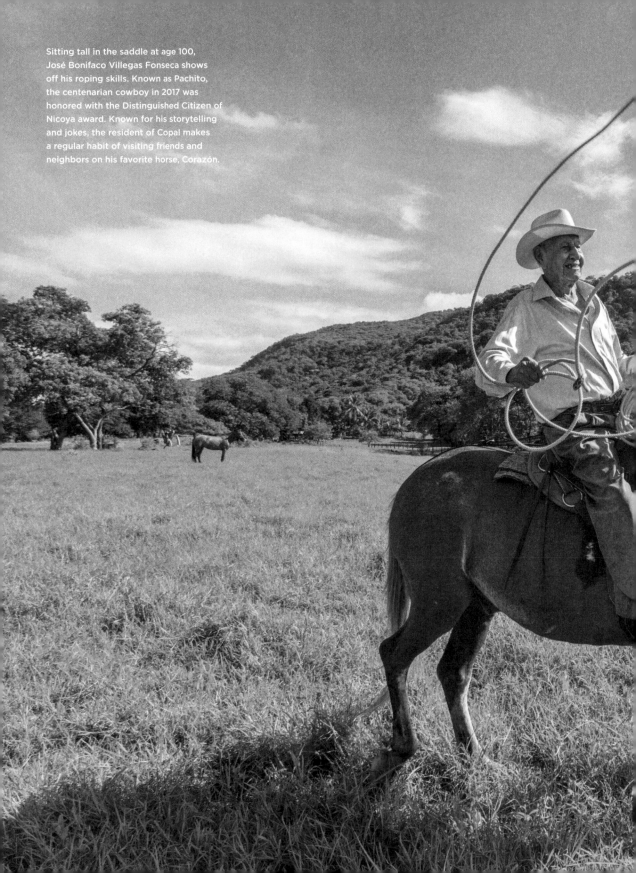

Sitting tall in the saddle at age 100, José Bonifaco Villegas Fonseca shows off his roping skills. Known as Pachito, the centenarian cowboy in 2017 was honored with the Distinguished Citizen of Nicoya award. Known for his storytelling and jokes, the resident of Copal makes a regular habit of visiting friends and neighbors on his favorite horse, Corazón.

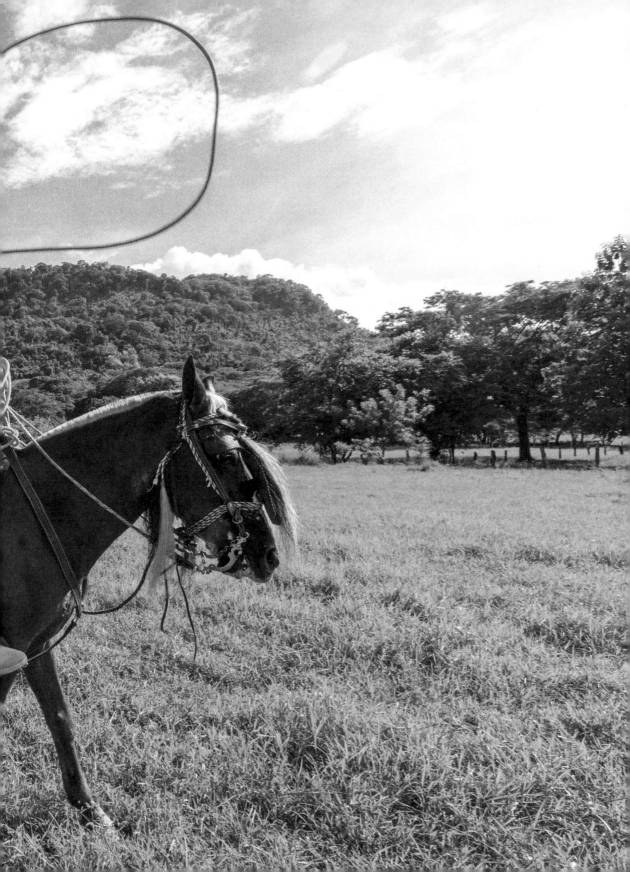

# Picadillo de Chayote
# (Veggie Hash With Corn and Onions)

**TOTAL COOK TIME: 25 MINUTES • SERVES 4**

Picadillo is the consummate Costa Rican comfort food and is popular throughout Latin America. It's similar to a potato hash, as all the ingredients are chopped into small pieces. The name comes from the Spanish word *picar,* which means "to chop." Costa Rican versions also include the names of the main vegetables involved, such as *picadillo de ayote* (squash) and *picadillo de palmito* (heart of palm).

*Picadillo de chayote* is an authentic and easy Costa Rican family dish, whether you enjoy it as a filling for tortillas or pair it with soup and rice to make a hearty meal.

1 large chayote squash, peeled, pitted, and diced

3 ears corn, kernels removed, or 1 cup frozen sweet corn kernels

3 sweet red or yellow peppers, seeded and diced

½ sweet onion (like Vidalia), minced

4 teaspoons chopped culantro or cilantro

1 celery stalk, diced

2 cloves garlic, minced

1 cup water

1 teaspoon achiote paste*

Salt and pepper (optional)

In a large pot or sauté pan, combine all ingredients. Cook over medium heat until there is a thick "gravy" at the bottom of the pan, about 15 to 20 minutes. Add salt and pepper, to taste, if using.

*Achiote paste is a cooking condiment used to add red color and a mild chili flavor to dishes. You can find it in Mexican or Latin markets or online. It is a mix of achiote and several other spices and is often sold as a spice cake. If you can't find it, you can use paprika or mild chili powder with a squeeze of lime.

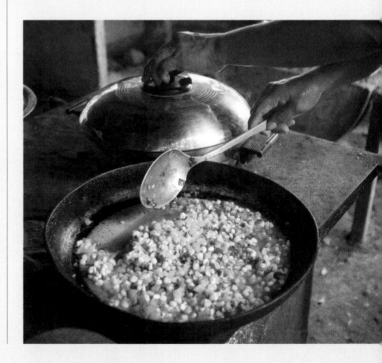

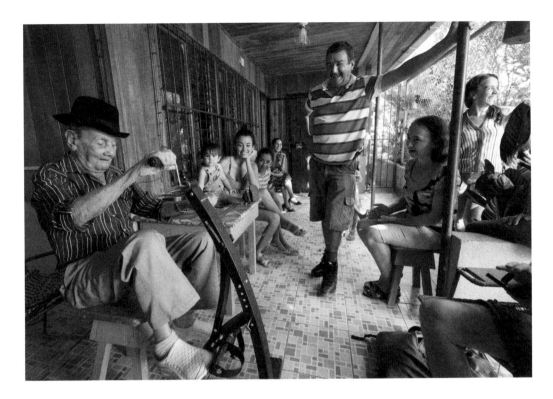

Saúl Guzmán Salas tries out an exercise machine on his porch in Hojancha as his family looks on.

I was accompanied by Álvaro Salas Chaves, the former head of Costa Rica's national health agency. Salas had spent a year in Nicoya in the late 1970s on a government-sponsored mobile health project, and it had made a lasting impression on him. "This was a very isolated place back then," he said. "People were quite poor."

After working his way up the ladder, Salas had led an effort in the 1990s to create a new rural health-care system. Under the program, called Equipos Básicos de Atención Integral en Salud (EBAIS), small teams were created, including a physician, a nurse, a record keeper, and a trained health worker. Each team was assigned a specific population to care for, with each household getting at least one visit per year. These teams became the frontline workers in Costa Rica's new campaign for preventive medicine.

"If you ask me, public health is responsible for 30 to 40 percent of Nicoya's longevity formula," Salas said. "Most of the people here don't need a surgeon. They need education, a clean water supply, and vaccines. They need a holistic approach."

As we chatted on the porch with Venerando, the growl of a motorcycle grew louder, and I turned to see a figure bounce up the dirt road. It was the local EBAIS worker paying the family a visit. After parking his bike, he came over with his backpack and introduced himself as Wesley Rafael Fonseca Dinarte. While he told us about his rounds—EBAIS workers visit as many as a dozen households a day—he took Venerando's blood pressure and asked him a few questions to screen him for depression.

Fonseca Dinarte clearly knew Venerando's health record, as he did that of all the residents he visited. As part of the organization's proactive approach, EBAIS keeps track of who has a chronic disease or a disability and who lives alone in their elderly years. He gave Venerando some anti-parasite medication, which he and Rosa take prophylactically. And in a gentle but firm tone, he told the old man that the cooking fire in their kitchen was bad for the couple's lungs and they should move it outside. Before he left, he did a quick search around the house for evidence of standing water in places where mosquitoes that carry malaria, dengue fever, or the Zika virus might breed. Then he returned to his motorcycle, which had a small cooler strapped onto the back containing a variety of vaccines, mostly for children.

Paulina Villegas serves a hearty breakfast to her centenarian father, José, and her nephew, Sixto.

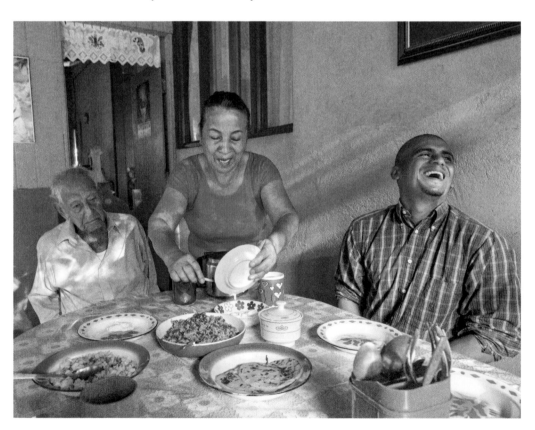

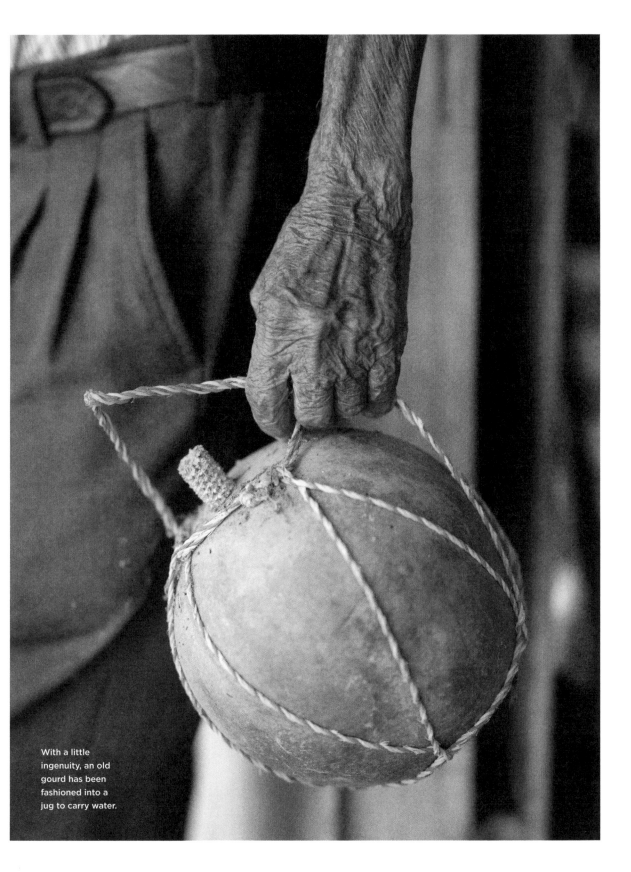

With a little ingenuity, an old gourd has been fashioned into a jug to carry water.

At a party to celebrate her 100th birthday, Jésús Dávila takes a spin around the dance floor with her son in the rural town of Belén in the Carrillo district. Nicoyans have a knack for enjoying life in the moment, an attitude captured by the expression *pura vida,* which means "all good" or "take it easy."

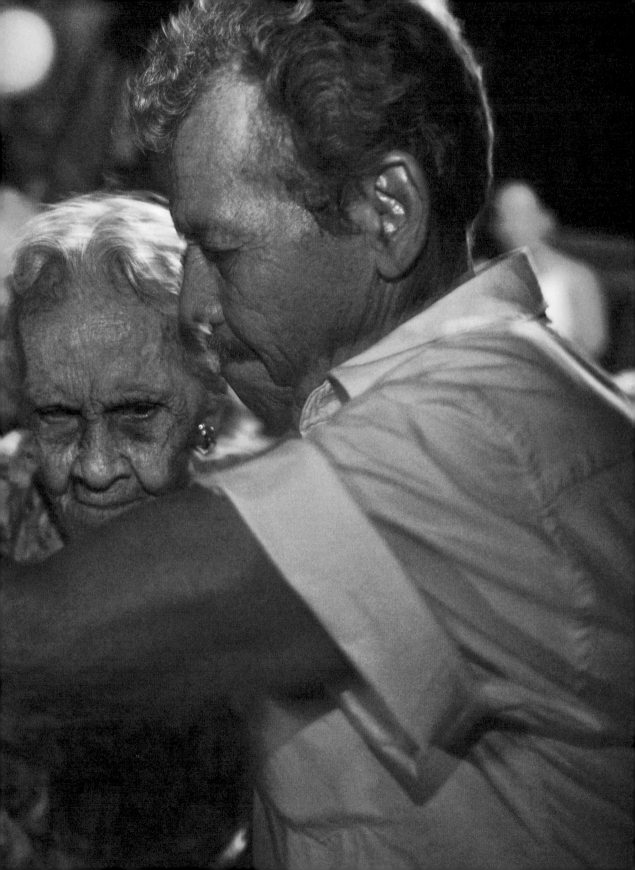

"What you've just seen is a hospital without walls," Salas said. "The idea is to reach people before they need a hospital. It's much cheaper and more effective."

The health-care movement that brought EBAIS to the countryside has

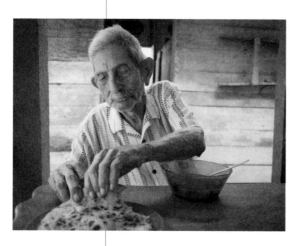

paid huge dividends for Costa Rica. Since EBAIS was started, deaths from communicable diseases have fallen by 94 percent, infant mortality has dropped by a factor of seven, and life expectancy has risen from 66 to 80 years. The politician responsible for promoting this movement was the same one who chose Salas to run the national health-care agency. His name is José María Figueres, and one afternoon in 2016 he waited for me at a Denny's restaurant in San José.

Known as Chepe to his friends, José María Guevara Pizarro, 108, digs into a simple lunch.

Figueres was seated by himself at a table in the middle of the dining room, nursing a cup of tea. A short, energetic-looking man, he wore a white guayabera shirt and loafers. A fringe of brown hair covered his otherwise smooth head. When I reached the table, he shook my hand, gave my arm a squeeze, and welcomed me to his country.

Figueres was only 39 when he was elected president in 1994 as the candidate of the center-left National Liberation Party. His father, José Figueres Ferrer, had led the revolution in 1948 that resulted in the founding of modern Costa Rica. Known as "Don Pepe" to the people, the elder Figueres was a social democrat who disbanded the army, granted full citizenship to women and Black

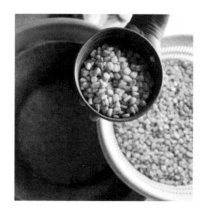

## NIXTAMAL

Before corn kernels can be ground and turned into tortillas, they are soaked and cooked in calcium hydroxide, or lime and water, and then washed and hulled. This process infuses the kernels with calcium and unlocks amino acids for the body to absorb. The resulting corn is then ready to be ground into *nixtamal*, also called masa harina. When paired with beans and rice, and topped with peppers, onions, and garlic, the corn tortillas wrap up a meal with complete nutrition for the day—one that's rich in calcium, protein, and niacin. Even so, the average Nicoyan still consumes 25 percent fewer calories than the average person in the United States.

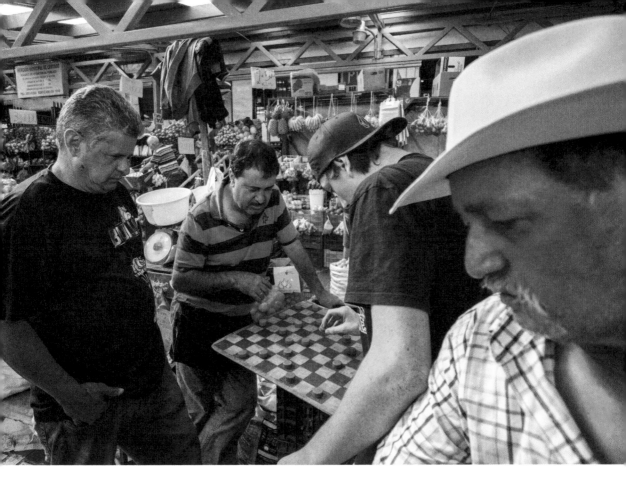

Costa Ricans, nationalized the banks, taxed the wealthy, and strengthened the nation's health-care and education systems during his three terms as president.

"My father was a self-taught man," Figueres told me. "He wanted to create government programs that would, in a way, level the playing field and open up opportunities for everybody."

As we chatted in the restaurant, people kept coming up to the table to thank the former president for his service to the country, and he seemed happy to greet them. "Costa Rica has a very egalitarian society in terms of our social behavior. Everybody talks to everybody else in this country," he said.

The EBAIS system was created in a similar egalitarian spirit—to extend the same quality of health care found in the cities to rural areas. "The whole idea of EBAIS, when we put it together 20 years ago, was to divide the Costa Rican map into little geographies, each one having between 2,500 and 4,000 inhabitants," Figueres said. "If you went inside one of the EBAIS clinics, you would find a red flag on this house, meaning that in this house you would find

Alejandro Zuñiga (left), known as Chamber, looks on as his fellow produce vendors play checkers in the municipal market in Cartago.

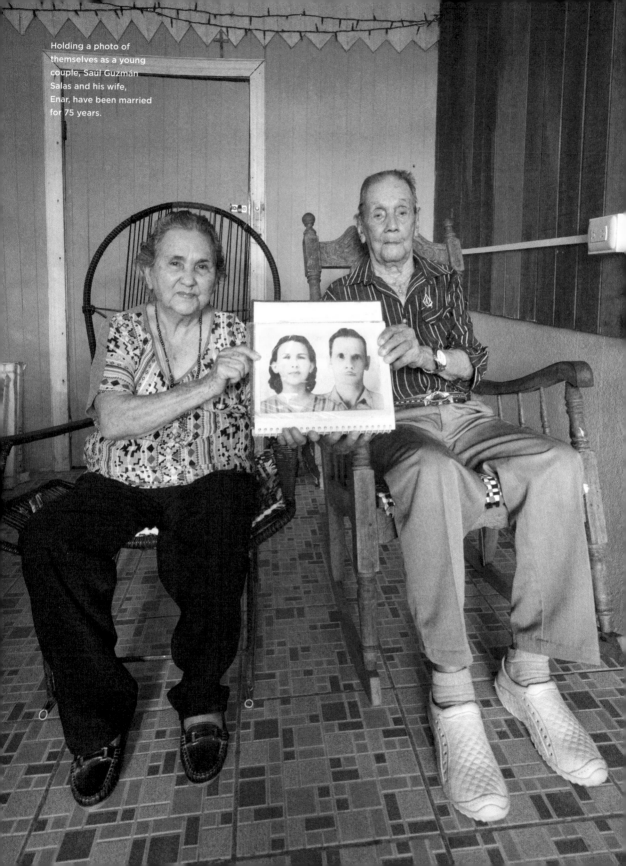

Holding a photo of themselves as a young couple, Saúl Guzmán Salas and his wife, Enar, have been married for 75 years.

someone with a coronary situation. And you would have a blue flag on this home, meaning this person has hypertension or high blood pressure. And you would find a yellow flag in this other home, meaning this person has diabetes. The whole objective was that these teams would take care of people who came to the EBAIS in the morning. And then in the afternoon they would go and visit, home by home, the community. Like your family doctor in the old days."

"Could a system like that work in the United States?" I asked.

"No," he replied. "Because your incentives are in the exact opposite direction. In the U.S., incentives are aligned to drive up costs, because when you increase costs, everybody wins—except the person who gets sick. Here, for years, the emphasis has been on the preventive health system, because, quite frankly, the objective of a good health policy is for people not to get sick. If we can prevent a cold in a 60-year-old person before it becomes pneumonia, then he won't have to go to the hospital at $1,500 per night."

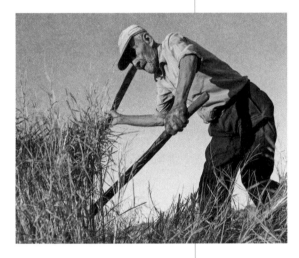

The work never ends for centenarians who live off the land.

I left my interview with Figueres feeling as if more pieces of the Costa Rican puzzle were coming together. There was the simple, plant-based diet of traditional Nicoyans; the lifelong work ethic of their eldest residents; their faith in God and their strong family bonds; and now the proactive health system that kept them out of the hospital.

Unfortunately, as Rosero-Bixby has recently calculated, the longevity phenomenon in Nicoya is rapidly disappearing. While Nicoyan men born before 1910 lived 6.4 years more than their fellow Costa Ricans, that advantage has shrunk to only half a year for men born in the 1940s. Not only that, the geographic area of the Nicoyan blue zone has also shrunk to a fraction of what it once was and is now restricted to an area bounded by the towns of Nosara and Samara Beach along the coast and Hojancha in the north. The larger towns on the peninsula are no longer part of the Nicoyan blue zone.

This should come as no surprise, I guess. The same forces that are eroding traditional lifestyles in places like Sardinia and Okinawa—new roads, communication, tourism, the invasion of junk food, and social media—are also at work in Nicoya. Under the banner of progress, the region's unique mix of hardship,

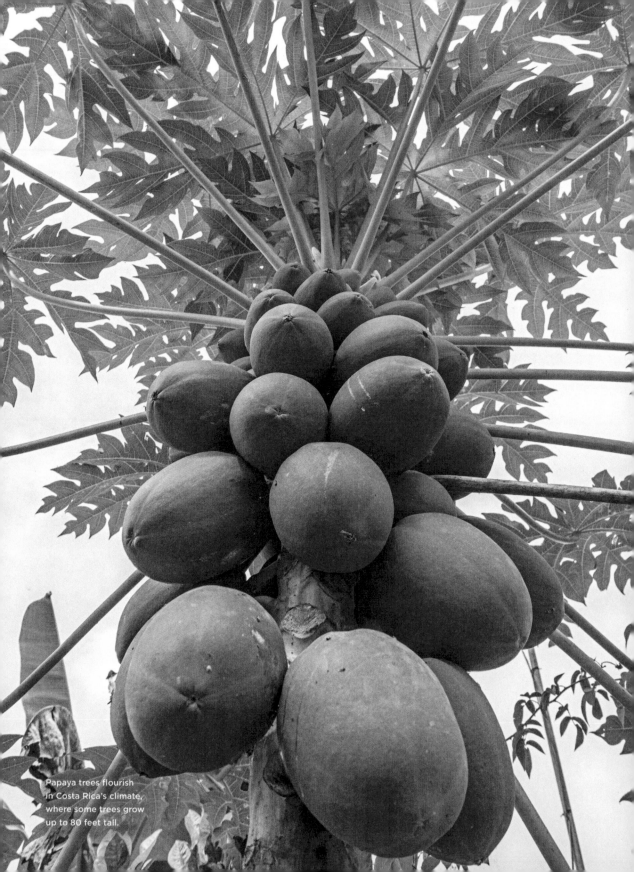

Papaya trees flourish in Costa Rica's climate, where some trees grow up to 80 feet tall.

# Top Longevity Foods From Nicoya

Among the favorites of the Costa Rican diet, corn and black beans stand out as superfoods. Corn tortillas provide complex carbohydrates loaded with vitamins, minerals, and fiber, while black beans contain more antioxidants than any other bean. Put together, they supply all the amino acids our bodies need to thrive. In Nicoya's traditional diet, about 80 percent of the daily calories came from different types of carbohydrates, including grains that add up to about 26 percent of their typical diet, with the remaining 20 percent of calories coming from various proteins and fats in about equal measure.

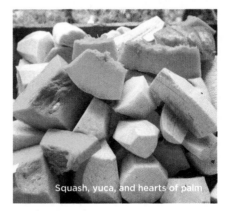
Squash, yuca, and hearts of palm

**SMALL SWEET PEPPERS** | Rich in vitamins, especially vitamin C, these peppers provide several health benefits, including reduced risk of a number of chronic diseases.

**BLACK BEANS** | Full of fiber and protein, black beans help reduce bad cholesterol and aid digestion.

**GROUND CORN** | Used to make tortillas, nixtamal is eaten at breakfast, lunch, and dinner. It increases the body's ability to absorb calcium, iron, and minerals.

**CILANTRO** | Used in many Nicoyan dishes, this herb is known to help lower blood sugar levels and reduce the risk of cardiovascular diseases. It also aids digestion.

**COCONUT** | A good source of healthy saturated fats that actually boost fat burning, coconut also increases HDL cholesterol (the good kind), which is linked to a lower risk of heart disease.

**CULANTRO** | Also known as Mexican coriander, culantro is related to cilantro but has a much stronger flavor. It is rich in calcium, iron, and riboflavin.

**CHILERO SAUCE** | Probably the most popular condiment in Costa Rica, chilero sauce gives a probiotic boost to dishes from its vinegar and antioxidant and antibacterial properties from its peppers.

**PAPAYA** | These trees grow almost like weeds in Nicoya. The rich, orange flesh of their fruit contains vitamins A, C, and E, plus papain, which counters inflammation.

**SQUASH** | Known for providing high levels of useful carotenoids, squash belongs to the botanical family Cucurbitaceae and is available in several varieties.

**YUCA** | Also known as cassava, yuca is a good source of vitamin C and antioxidants. Basically, it's a powerhouse for boosting immunity and fighting infections and viruses.

hard work, faith, family ties, and a healthy diet is getting shredded in the cultural blender.

But not everywhere in Nicoya yet.

Back at Don Ramiro's house south of Santa Cruz, the centenarian was holding court with his granddaughters, Melisa, 30, and Krisia, 22, and his great-grandson Isaac, 4. As they sat under a wooden canopy in his backyard, a couple of chickens scooted past. He gestured at his family and smiled.

"This is why I'm still here," he said. "They make me happy."

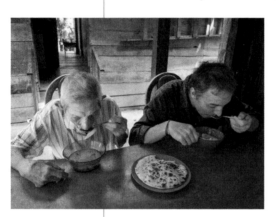

Below: Chepe Guevara, 106, eats with Dan.

Later, when it cooled off and his family went back home, he planned to chop some wood for his cooking fire, or maybe prepare a little food for later. Then in late afternoon, when the sun was lower in the sky, he'd get back on his horse and return to his cattle to move them one more time and make sure they had water.

On his way to the farm, he might make a detour through the village to pass by the house of a young woman he found attractive, he said. With any luck, she'd be sitting on her porch, and he could give her a little wave as he rode by.

"If the eyes don't see, the heart doesn't feel," he told me. Which I took to mean, "if you stop looking, you stop living."

Since his wife died many years ago, Don Ramiro has had seven *novías* (girlfriends), he said. Once in a blue moon, he might drop by a village bar and treat himself to a glass of Johnnie Walker Black. Sometimes he'd dance.

Could this be another secret to his longevity?

I recalled what Rosero-Bixby had told me on our first visit to Nicoya. We'd been discussing mortality rates and survey data and other academic topics, and I'd asked him if there was anything else that might explain what kept men alive so long in this region.

He was driving at the time, and he threw me a side glance. "You know, in Latin America we take marriage very seriously. If you get married, there's great pressure to stay married your whole life. But here …" He hesitated. "Well, men here have very liberated attitudes toward sex. They tend to have many sexual partners throughout life."

Sex and longevity? That was a new one.

Opposite (clockwise from top left): "We eat what God provides," says María Norberta Marchena Díaz, 107. In Nicoya, that often means black beans, white sweet potatoes, and other vegetables. A strong faith tradition also supports long life.

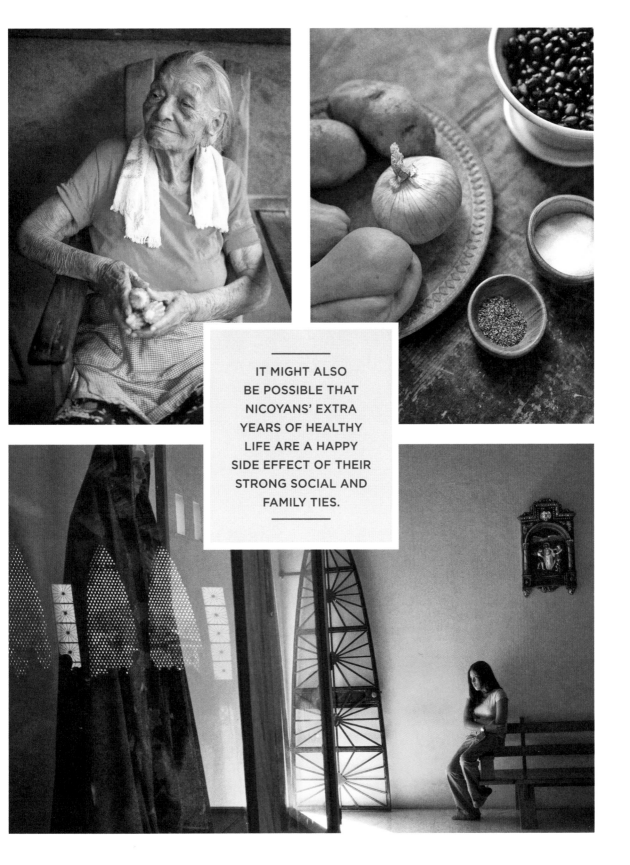

IT MIGHT ALSO BE POSSIBLE THAT NICOYANS' EXTRA YEARS OF HEALTHY LIFE ARE A HAPPY SIDE EFFECT OF THEIR STRONG SOCIAL AND FAMILY TIES.

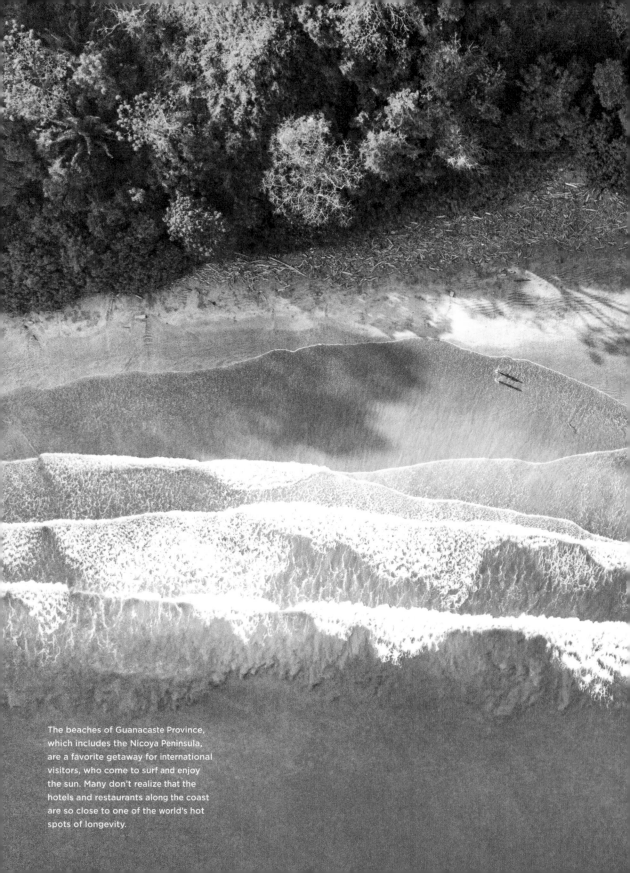

The beaches of Guanacaste Province, which includes the Nicoya Peninsula, are a favorite getaway for international visitors, who come to surf and enjoy the sun. Many don't realize that the hotels and restaurants along the coast are so close to one of the world's hot spots of longevity.

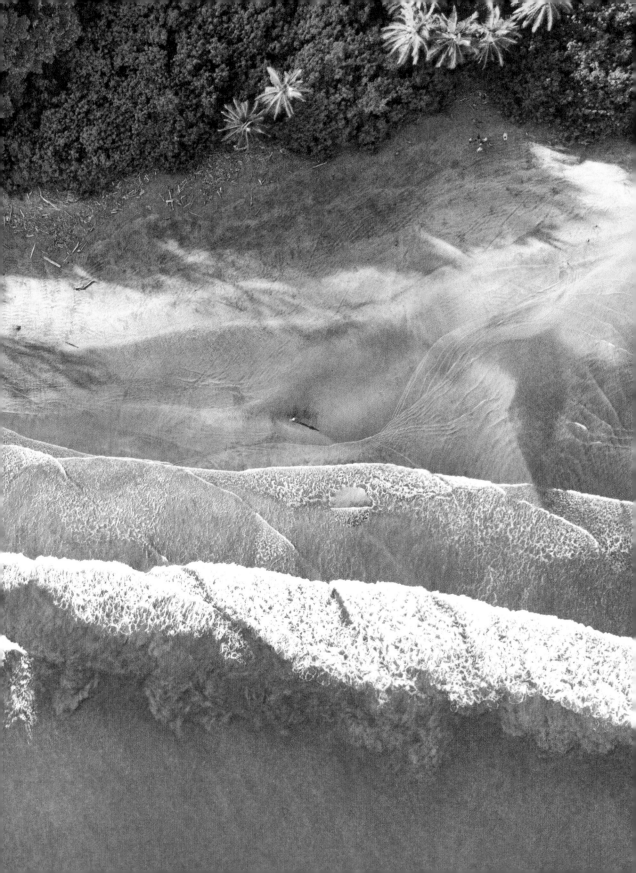

# LESSONS FROM COSTA RICA'S BLUE ZONE

■ **Have a *plan de vida***

Successful centenarians have a strong sense of purpose. They feel needed and want to contribute to a greater good.

■ **Drink hard water**

Nicoyan water has the country's highest calcium content, perhaps explaining the lower rates of heart disease, as well as the stronger bones and fewer hip fractures.

■ **Keep a focus on family**

Nicoyan centenarians tend to live with their families, and children or grandchildren provide support and a sense of purpose and belonging.

■ **Eat a light dinner**

Eating fewer calories appears to be one of the surest ways to add years to your life. Nicoyans eat a light dinner early in the evening. Nicoyan centenarians ate a traditional Mesoamerican diet highlighted by the "three sisters" of agriculture: beans, corn, and squash.

■ **Maintain a social network**

Nicoyan centenarians get frequent visits from neighbors. They know how to listen, laugh, and appreciate what they have.

■ **Keep hard at work**

Centenarians seem to have enjoyed physical work all their lives. They find joy in everyday physical chores, including gardening, maintaining their land, cooking, and caring for their grandchildren.

■ **Get some sensible sun**

Nicoyans regularly take in the sunshine, which helps their bodies produce vitamin D for strong bones and healthy body function. Vitamin D deficiency is associated with a host of problems, such as osteoporosis and heart disease, but regular "smart" sun exposure (about 15 minutes on the legs and arms) can help supplement your diet and ensure you're getting enough of this vital nutrient.

■ **Embrace a common history**

Modern Nicoyans' roots to the Indigenous Chorotega and their traditions have enabled them to remain relatively free of stress. Their traditional diet of fortified maize and beans may be the best nutritional combination for longevity the world has ever known.

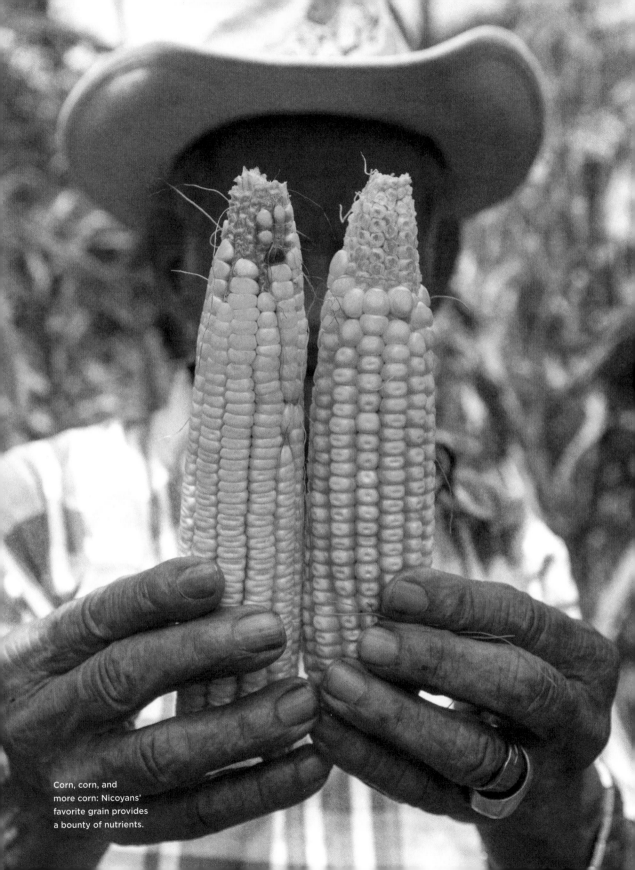

Corn, corn, and more corn: Nicoyans' favorite grain provides a bounty of nutrients.

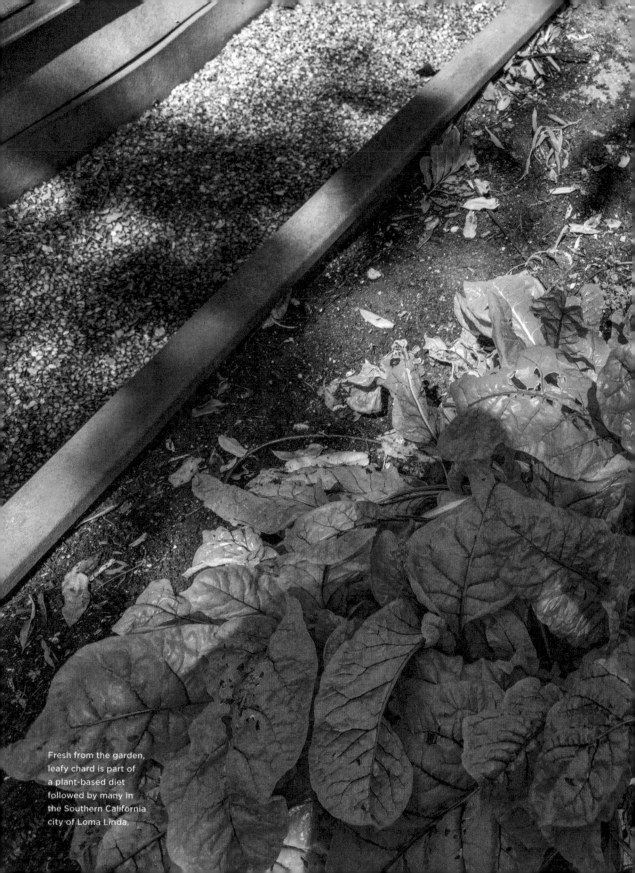

Fresh from the garden, leafy chard is part of a plant-based diet followed by many in the Southern California city of Loma Linda.

CHAPTER 3

# Loma Linda

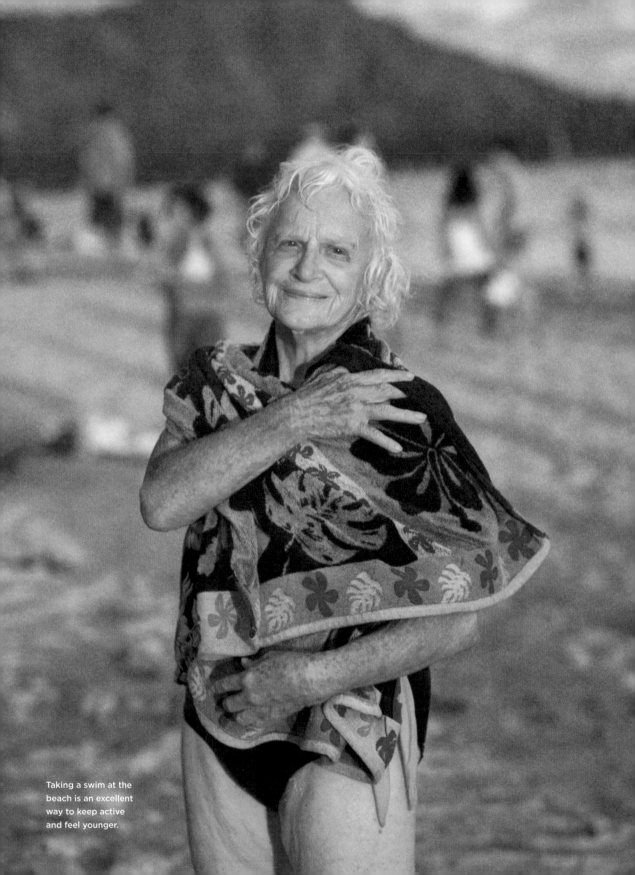

Taking a swim at the beach is an excellent way to keep active and feel younger.

# American Blue Zone

Sixty miles east of Los Angeles in the smog-ridden suburbs of the San Bernardino Valley, a community of about 9,000 Seventh-day Adventists defies the longevity odds. They represent some 20 million Adventists nationwide who live up to a decade longer than the rest of us. The Adventists credit their longevity to eight "natural remedies": pure air, sunlight, abstemiousness, rest, exercise, a plant-based diet, drinking water, and trust in divine power. And they back up their claims with data. Since the 1970s, Adventists who live in and around the city of Loma Linda have participated in health and diet studies that show they live longer than other Californians—7.3 years longer for men and 4.4 years longer for women. Vegetarian Adventists live 9.5 years longer for men and 6.1 years longer for women.

So, how exactly do they do it?

That was the question on my mind back in 2005 when I first drove to the city of Loma Linda from Los Angeles International Airport. As I barreled east down Interstate 10, I gazed at the mustard-colored haze draped over the San Bernardino Mountains to the north and the strip malls to the south. Taking the exit for Loma Linda, I passed through a gauntlet of fast-food franchises hawking fried chicken, tacos, burgers, french fries, sodas, and subs, which made me

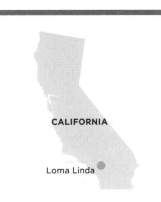

**CALIFORNIA**

Loma Linda

- Loma Linda, California, is home to a community of Seventh-day Adventists.

- The city is located in the sprawling suburbs of San Bernardino County.

- Many Seventh-day Adventists follow a plant-based diet.

- Adventists live an average of a decade longer than other Americans.

wonder if this small patch of suburbia could really be America's answer to Sardinia and Nicoya.

I was eager to meet Dr. Gary Fraser, the principal investigator of the Adventist Health Studies, a series of research projects that tracked the health of tens of thousands of Adventists for decades. After steadily climbing up the road (*loma linda* is Spanish for "lovely hill") to Loma Linda University Medical

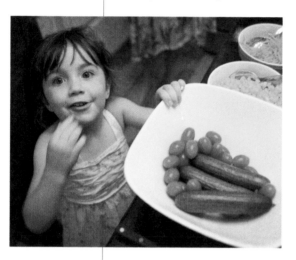

Fresh cherry tomatoes tempt a young girl to sneak a bite before dinner.

Center, I found Fraser's office in the sprawling campus of manicured lawns and six different hospitals that employ more than 900 physicians.

A native of New Zealand, Fraser struck me as a genial scoutmaster, with his neatly combed sandy brown hair. He'd started out as a cardiologist but had been frustrated by patients who'd neglected their bodies for years. "It was like trying to close the door to the barn after the horse has bolted," he said. "I decided to become an epidemiologist and see if I could help ward off heart disease on the front end, which is much more satisfying."

The university's first major health study, Adventist Health Study-1 (AHS-1), had been funded by the National Institutes of Health and ran from 1974 to 1988. Observing 34,000 Adventists in California, it produced some intriguing results. As expected, the researchers found that Adventists, who are mostly nonsmoking, had a 70 percent lower rate of lung cancer compared to non-Adventists. They also found that individuals who regularly got their fiber from fruits, vegetables, and grains reduced their risk of colon cancer by 40 percent, while those who ate meat several times a week increased theirs by 60 percent. Not only that, but the researchers also found that eating nuts several times a week cut one's risk of suffering a heart attack by up to 50 percent.

"Clearly, a plant-based diet is the way to go," Fraser said.

In the spring of 2021, I caught up with him again by phone to discuss the results of a second, larger study, Adventist Health Study-2, which began in 2002 and continues to this day.

"It's a powerful study design," he said of the ongoing project funded by the National Cancer Institute and National Institutes of Health. About 96,000 participants are grouped into four categories: vegans, lacto-ovo vegetarians (those who consume dairy and eggs), pesco-vegetarians (those who eat fish and very little meat), and nonvegetarians. "Some live one way, some live another. We said, let's follow them over time and find out how their health experiences compare."

As the new study confirmed, strict vegetarian Adventists can expect to live nearly a decade longer than other Americans, with a fraction of their chronic diseases and cancers. In particular, the researchers calculated that a vegetarian diet reduces one's risk of developing type 2 diabetes by 50 percent and coronary heart disease by 60 percent. By contrast, Adventists who regularly eat meat have a 46 percent higher rate of premature death than those who get their protein from nuts, seeds, and legumes. The meat eaters also tend to weigh about 20 pounds more than the vegetarians.

Although vegan participants are more likely to weigh less than others in the study, they don't live the longest, the researchers found. That distinction went to pesco-vegetarians, those who eat up to one serving of fish per day in addition to their regular plant-based diet.

Everyone in the family pitches in to make dinner, which includes a platter of fresh fruits.

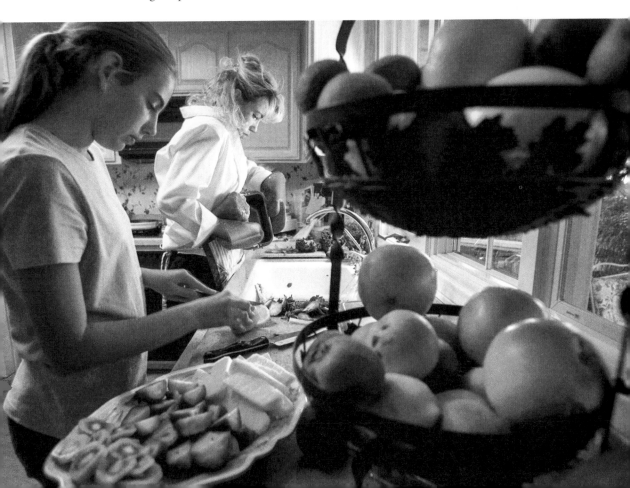

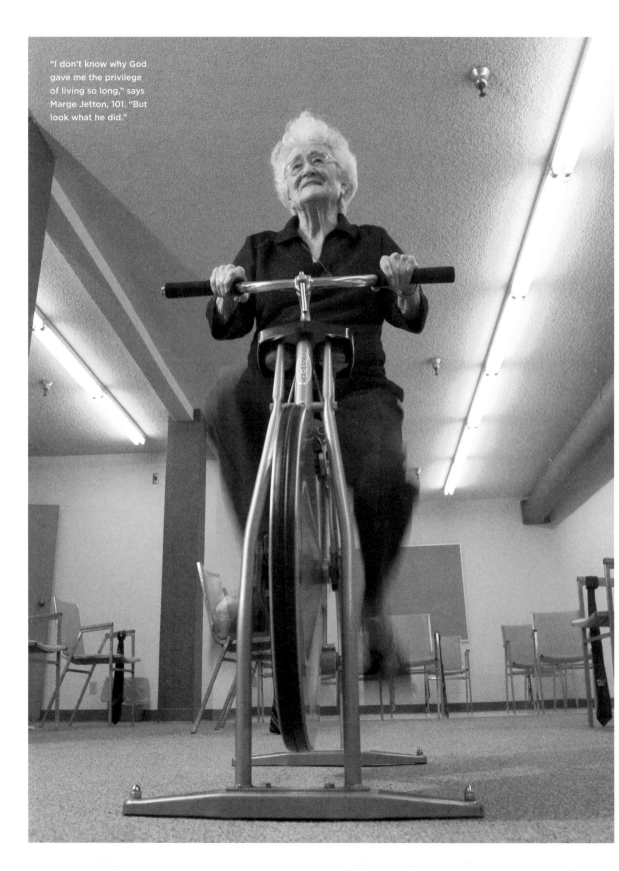

"I don't know why God gave me the privilege of living so long," says Marge Jetton, 101. "But look what he did."

Fraser and his team also discovered an alarming connection between milk and two types of cancer. Men who consume roughly 1¾ cups of milk per day face a 25 percent greater chance of developing prostate cancer, they learned, while women who consume as little as ¼ cup of milk face a 30 percent greater chance of developing breast cancer. One possible reason for this increased risk might be the hormones in milk from pregnant cows, since breast cancer in women has been shown to be hormone responsive.

"So, what does it all mean if we want to live longer?" I asked.

"It's not that complicated," Fraser replied. "I don't think there's any secret to what Adventists are doing. We've just found a way to put it into practice."

All you need to do is follow as many of these practices as possible, he said:

1) Eat a vegetarian diet. That will earn you an extra two years of life.

2) Get regular exercise because it's good for your heart.

3) Don't smoke—it's a leading cause of lung cancer and heart disease.

4) Be careful with your body weight. It has a huge impact on cardiovascular disease, blood pressure, cholesterol, and inflammation.

5) Snack on nuts. Nuts protect your heart and add another two years to your life.

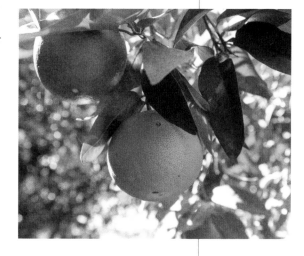

Loma Linda Adventists value fresh produce, including oranges, which grow abundantly in local groves.

Participants of the Adventist study who did all five of these things got the full 10-year boost in their life expectancy, Fraser said. And they not only lived longer; they also lived *better*.

As I drove around Loma Linda in the winter of 2021, I was astounded to see how little the community had changed since my first visit. Except for some new buildings at the university, it looked just like it had 17 years ago, with its quiet neighborhoods and neatly manicured lawns sloping up the hill from the medical center. The Wiener Hut across from the main hospital was gone, I noticed, replaced by a Carl's Jr. But the Loma Linda Market was still there, with aisle after aisle of organic foods and more than 80 bins of seeds and nuts. As large as most national chain grocery stores, it offered customers soy-based vegan jerky, "Fishless Sticks," and egg-free ice cream. Except for the new juice bar, it looked the same as ever.

I probably shouldn't have been surprised. By their nature, Seventh-day

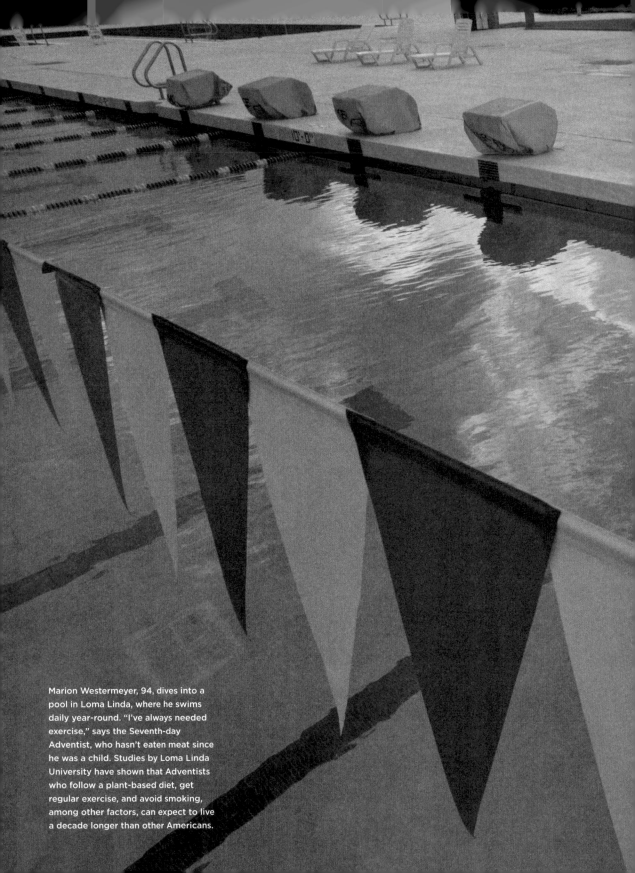

Marion Westermeyer, 94, dives into a pool in Loma Linda, where he swims daily year-round. "I've always needed exercise," says the Seventh-day Adventist, who hasn't eaten meat since he was a child. Studies by Loma Linda University have shown that Adventists who follow a plant-based diet, get regular exercise, and avoid smoking, among other factors, can expect to live a decade longer than other Americans.

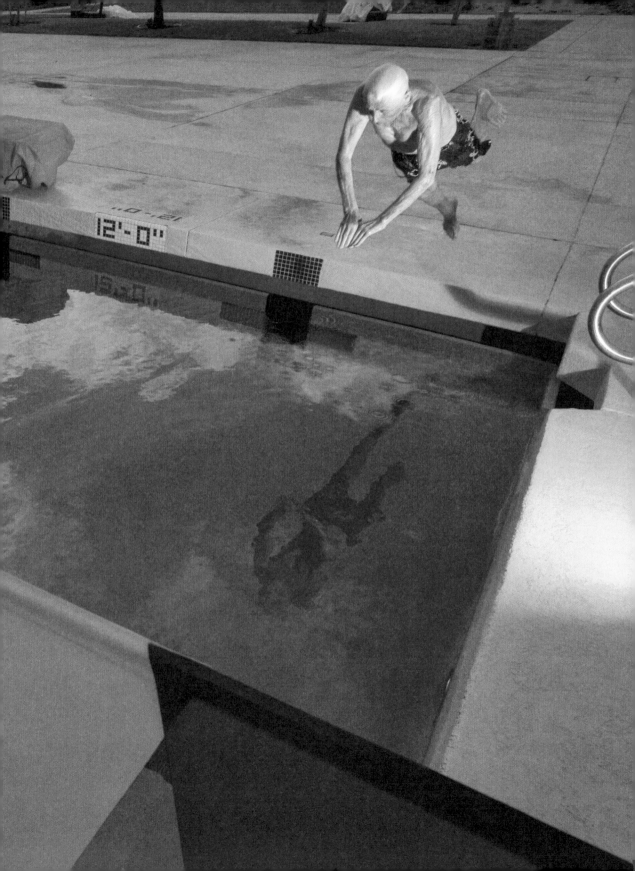

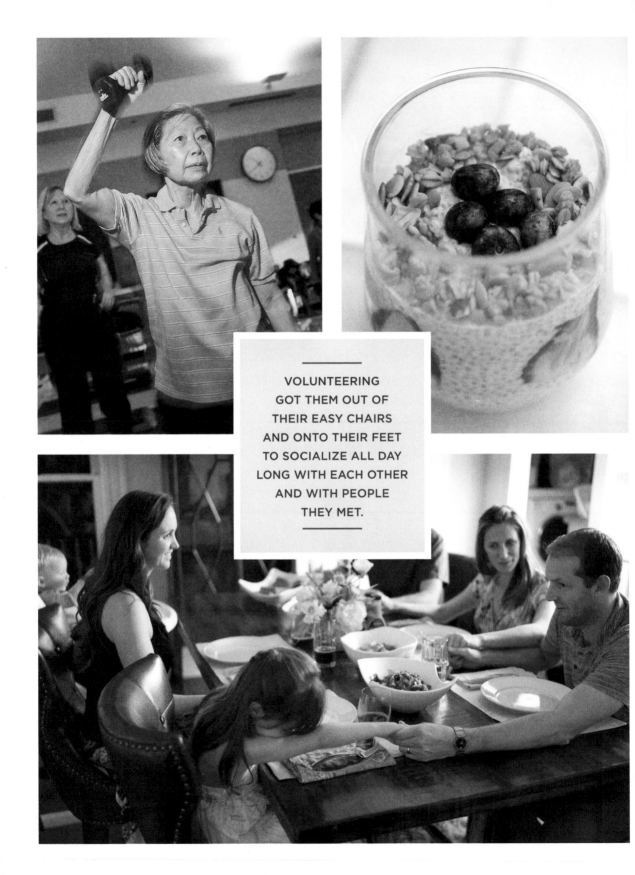

VOLUNTEERING
GOT THEM OUT OF
THEIR EASY CHAIRS
AND ONTO THEIR FEET
TO SOCIALIZE ALL DAY
LONG WITH EACH OTHER
AND WITH PEOPLE
THEY MET.

Adventists tend to be a conservative bunch. Their church, officially founded in 1860, grew out of the Second Great Awakening, a Protestant revival movement that promoted frontier-style camp meetings, Bible study, evangelism, and personal salvation. A few of the church's early leaders advocated giving up smoking, alcohol, meat, coffee, tea, and spices even before it became part of church doctrine. Today, some of the most conservative Adventists still don't believe in going to the movies or the theater or indulging in any form of popular culture.

That may be part of the secret to their success. Unlike other blue zones like Okinawa or Nicoya, where traditional lifestyles are fast disappearing, this California community has found a way to weather the winds of change. By offering a bulwark against the temptations of the world, the Seventh-day Adventist Church makes it easier for its members to stay on the straight and narrow.

I met a few foot soldiers in the local campaign to save souls one chilly morning as they prepared to spread the word from a suburban garage. Paul Demazo, 96, helped organize the Loma Linda chapter of the Volunteers of the Literature Ministry. He was joined on this bright February day by Gary Gifford, Carl Schwelt, and Terry Ingram.

The Literature Ministry dates back 100 years or so, Demazo told me. The Adventists have a long history of distributing literature to reinforce their beliefs and spread the word, and these guys were part of a team. One went around the community and persuaded doctors' offices and other businesses to let them put up racks for pamphlets, books, and magazines such as *Signs of the Times*. The others made the

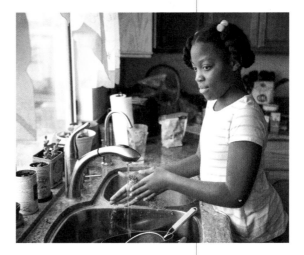

rounds to ensure the racks were kept filled. The garage I met them in was filled with boxes of inventory.

As part of the Literature Ministry, these four men, the youngest of whom was 80, were doing their part to spread their faith. But, I noted, their volunteering got them out of their easy chairs and onto their feet to socialize all day long with each other and with people they met. Plus, their commitment to help the church made them happy.

Opposite (clockwise from top left): Exercise at the community center, healthy foods like coconut chia pudding, and family bonds contribute to the longevity of Adventists in Loma Linda.

Above: Matea Brooks rinses off herbs in the kitchen for a family meal.

Demazo was a big fan of the need to stay active. "I had a huge group of friends that retired at age 65," he said. "We buried a third of them the first year."

When I asked him for his secret to having so much energy at 96, he referred

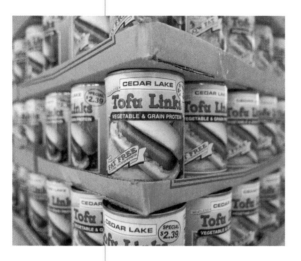

me to the eight natural remedies, revealed in a prophecy to Ellen G. White, one of the founders of the Seventh-day Adventist Church. White had championed the idea that taking care of your body was a religious duty. In her 1905 book, *The Ministry of Healing,* she defined nature's remedies as pure air, sunlight, abstemiousness, rest, exercise, proper diet, the use of water, and trust in divine power. "Every person should have a knowledge of nature's remedial agencies and how to apply them. It is essential both to understand the principles involved in the treatment of the sick and to have a practical training that will enable one rightly to use this knowledge," she wrote.

Meatless items are popular in Loma Linda's supermarkets, with aisle after aisle of organic foods and bins of seeds and nuts.

White put her theory into practice in 1866 by helping establish the Western Health Form Institute, a hydrotherapy clinic in Battle Creek, Michigan, where she and her husband, James, had moved their family. Convinced that the clinic needed a true medical professional at the helm, she recruited a young Adventist named James Harvey Kellogg to attend medical school at the University of Michigan. When he returned to Battle Creek in 1876, Kellogg shifted the focus of the clinic from water cures to preventive medicine based on a combination of Adventist-style diet and exercise and the latest medical and

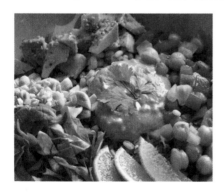

## GRAIN BOWLS

Easy to make, easy to store, and easy to eat, heavenly grain bowls are a convenient way to combine heart-healthy grains, beans, greens, and veggies into an appetizing meal. For grains, choose from brown rice, farro, couscous, quinoa, or wheat berries. Black beans, lentils, kidney beans, and cannellini beans add richness, while lettuce, kale, spinach, zucchini, and tomatoes add zing. Top with sliced avocados, sprouts, herbs, crushed nuts, seeds, or fried shallots, and dress with sriracha, honey mustard, lemon vinaigrette, pesto, harissa, or salsa.

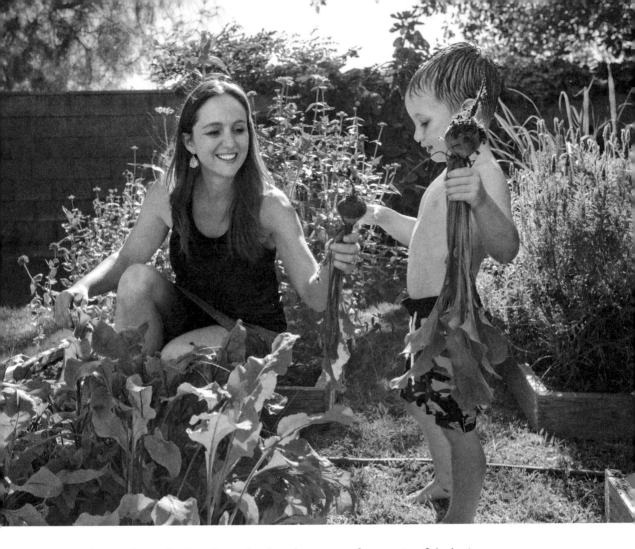

surgical procedures. (Kellogg later developed a process for creating flaked cereal with his brother, W. K. Kellogg, who formed the Battle Creek Toasted Corn Flake Company in 1906.) Today, there are 168 Adventists hospitals around the world.

White's prescriptions for healthy living seem remarkably prescient, mirroring guidelines from the American Cancer Society, the American Heart Association, and Harvard University's Healthy Eating Plate program. In her book *Counsels on Diet and Foods,* she wrote that "grains, fruits, nuts, and vegetables constitute the diet chosen for us by our Creator. These foods, prepared in as simple and natural a manner as possible, are the most healthful and nourishing. They impart a strength, a power of endurance, and a vigor of intellect that are not afforded by a more complex and stimulating diet." While discouraging the consumption of coffee and alcohol, she also warned against cooking with grease,

Three-year-old Austin Gheen helps his mother, Krystal, harvest beets from the family garden.

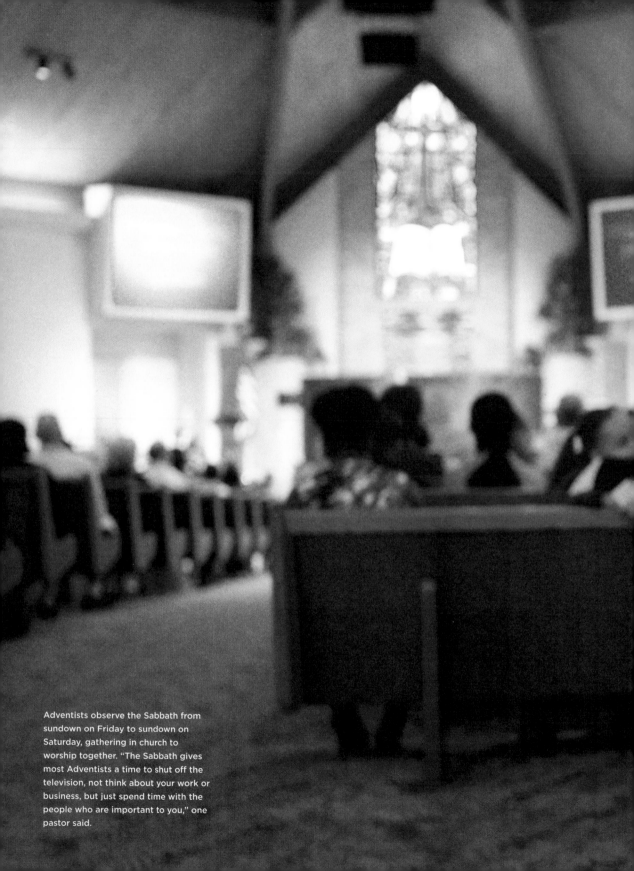

Adventists observe the Sabbath from sundown on Friday to sundown on Saturday, gathering in church to worship together. "The Sabbath gives most Adventists a time to shut off the television, not think about your work or business, but just spend time with the people who are important to you," one pastor said.

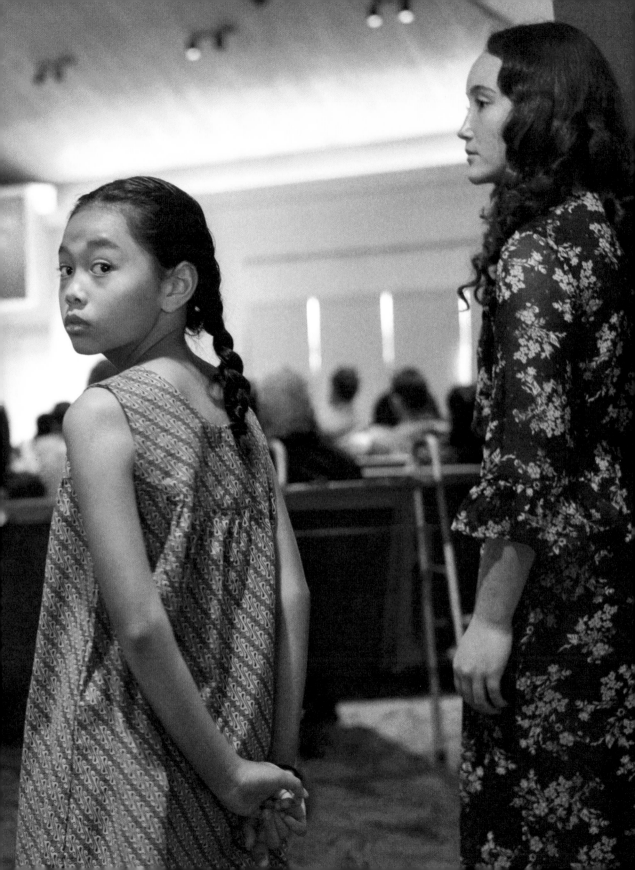

# Roasted Potatoes and Green Beans With Mustard Drizzle

TOTAL COOK TIME: 45 MINUTES • SERVES 4

In this deceptively simple recipe, the mustard dressing brightens all the flavors of this dish to create a spectacular one-pan meal. With beans, greens, and potatoes, it combines many of the most important staple foods from the blue zones.

**For the Roasted Vegetables:**

½ pound fingerling potatoes

3 garlic cloves, sliced

3 tablespoons chopped fresh parsley or other herbs

2 tablespoons extra-virgin olive oil

½ cup cooked chickpeas (or canned, drained, and rinsed), patted dry with a paper towel

½ pound green beans, washed, trimmed, and dried

**For the Dressing:**

1 tablespoon Dijon mustard

1½ tablespoons extra-virgin olive oil

1 tablespoon white wine vinegar

2 teaspoons honey

Salt and pepper (optional)

Heat your oven to 425°F.

In a large mixing bowl, toss the potatoes with the garlic, herbs, and olive oil.

Place the potatoes in a single layer in a roasting pan and roast for 25 minutes, or until fork-tender, stirring once or twice.

Add the chickpeas and green beans to the potatoes and roast for another 10 minutes.

While the vegetables roast, in a small bowl, whisk together the mustard, olive oil, vinegar, and honey to form an emulsified dressing.

Season the dressing with salt and pepper to taste.

Transfer the roasted vegetables and beans to a platter and drizzle with dressing. Serve warm.

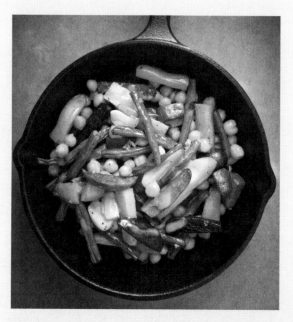

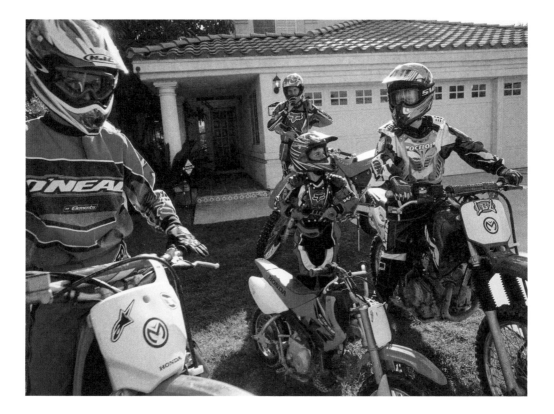

spices, and salt, among other things, and the use of sugar, which "causes fermentation and this clouds the brain and brings peevishness into the disposition."

To learn more about the science behind the Adventist diet, I met with Dr. Joan Sabaté, chair of Loma Linda University's Department of Nutrition. A native of Spain, he wore a subtle polka-dot shirt, a blue sports jacket, and flashy cobalt shoes when he greeted me in his office. As the principal architect of the vegetarian food guide pyramid, Sabaté has helped popularize the idea that a plant-based diet offers unique health benefits. With Gary Fraser and several colleagues, he authored a 1993 study showing that a diet that included walnuts as a snack, mixed in salads and breakfast cereals, or cooked in dinner entrées could lower serum cholesterol levels in men by more than 10 percent.

"Some people think that a vegetarian diet is just the absence of meat," he said. "But if you eat a variety of plant foods such as whole grains, legumes and soy, vegetables, fruits, and nuts and seeds, and get regular exercise, it can actually be protective. Eating beans, for example, often reduces the risk of colon cancer, even for meat eaters."

The Rawson family of Colton, California, prepare to go for a spin on their dirt bikes.

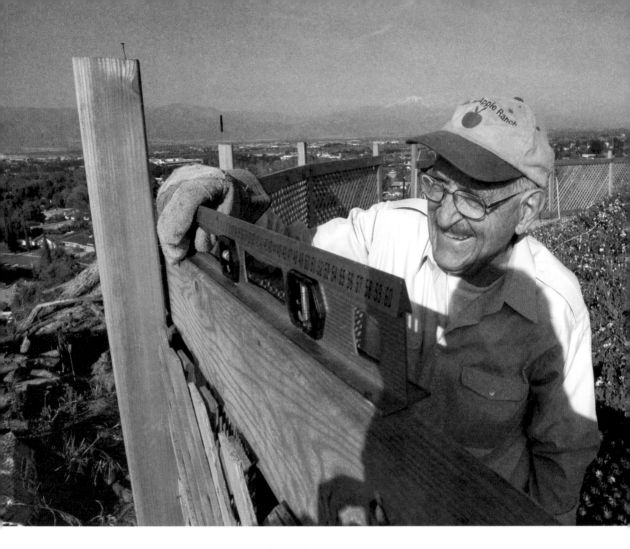

Retired heart surgeon Ellsworth Wareham, 91, builds a fence on the hillside behind his home.

It's easy to forget, he reminded me, given the popularity of the Mediterranean diet and other plant-based foods today, that people not so long ago believed that a diet without meat couldn't provide enough nutrients to stay healthy. But as the Adventist Health Studies have proved over the years, almost the opposite is true. Whole grains have been shown to prevent cardiovascular disease and colon cancer. Nuts have been shown to protect against heart disease. Plant-based diets in general boost one's immune system and increase life expectancy. The list goes on.

As an Adventist himself, Sabaté was careful to point out that the greater longevity of his community was due to more factors than a healthy diet. It also came from their entire lifestyle, which includes staying active, not smoking, keeping the Sabbath as a day of rest, and trusting in God. I'd learned about the Adventist Sabbath during my earlier visits to Loma Linda. Unlike most

Protestant denominations, which attend church on Sunday, the Adventists observe the Sabbath from sunset on Friday until sunset on Saturday. After going to church on Saturday, they get together with other Adventists for potluck lunches, or head out with friends or family for a hike or other activity outdoors.

The goal is to create a "sanctuary in time" when they can engage in quiet contemplation free from normal obligations—the "rest" that Ellen White prescribed as one of the essential remedies of nature.

As for the last factor on Sabaté's list— the importance of faith—I got a refresher course from a retired professor of religion at his home on a quiet cul-de-sac not far from the university. Dr. David Taylor stood in front of the open door to his garage, where he said he did his thinking and writing. There was no car or truck in there, just shelves filled with books and other religious publications.

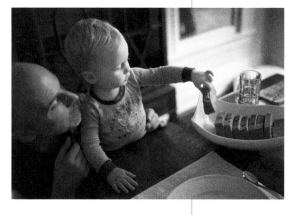

A toddler takes a slice of savory walnut "meat" loaf made with oats, breadcrumbs, and walnuts, but no meat.

"Why are all your books in the garage?" I asked. "Did your wife send you out here?"

He laughed. "No room inside. I needed a place to prepare for my classes and to speak to different groups. I like to keep the old brain supple."

"How old are you, if I may ask?"

"I'll be 89 in June," he replied.

Taylor and his wife, Maxine, came to Loma Linda in 1995 to teach at the university, he in the Department of Religion, she in the School of Allied Health. At the time, they were among the few Black professors on the staff.

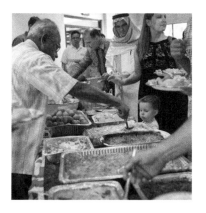

### THE SABBATH POTLUCK

A longtime tradition of the Adventist community, here and elsewhere around the country, the Sabbath potluck brings members of the Azure Hills Church together for a community meal. Some of the most popular foods that Loma Linda families bring to share with one another at such occasions are vegetarian gumbo, a taco salad known as "haystacks," no-meat meatballs, and various types of nut loaves. Besides attending church on the Sabbath, Adventists also spend the day getting together with family and friends, engaging in charitable works, and communing with nature by going on hikes, riding bikes, or taking a walk in a nearby park.

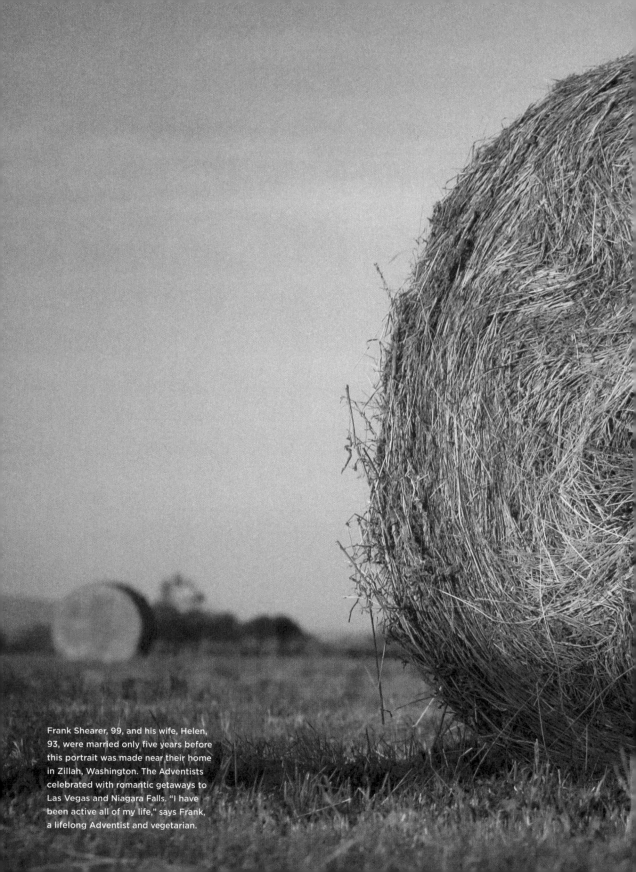

Frank Shearer, 99, and his wife, Helen, 93, were married only five years before this portrait was made near their home in Zillah, Washington. The Adventists celebrated with romantic getaways to Las Vegas and Niagara Falls. "I have been active all of my life," says Frank, a lifelong Adventist and vegetarian.

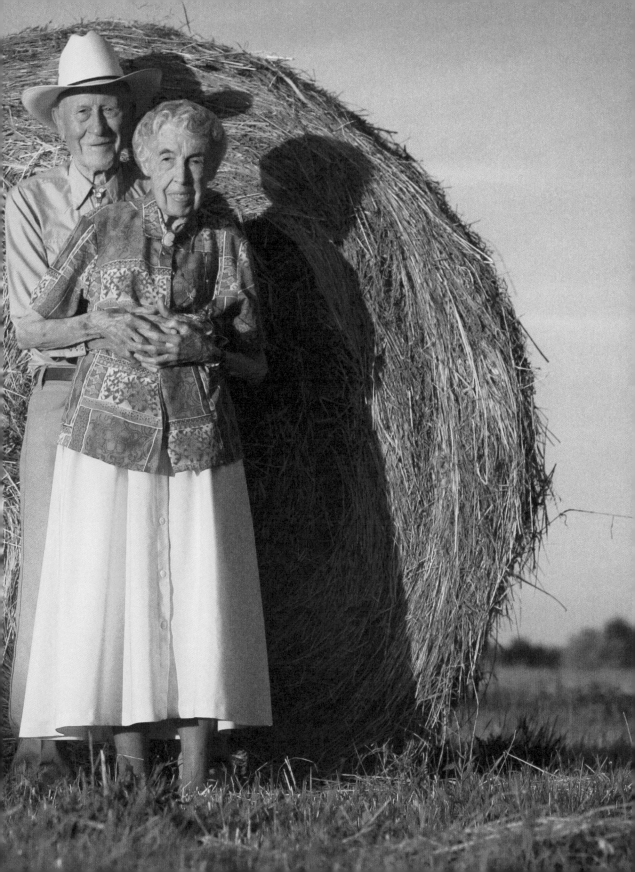

After a little prompting, he told me about his time at Oakwood College, a historically Black school owned by the Adventist church in Huntsville, Alabama. In March 1956, he and a group of classmates had driven to Montgomery to show their support for the Reverend Dr. Martin Luther King, Jr. during the protests that had followed the arrest of Rosa Parks the previous December. King had been indicted for his role in the bus boycott in Montgomery, and Taylor had managed to get a seat inside the courthouse for the trial.

As King entered the courtroom, he happened to notice Taylor sitting up front and asked the young man where he was from. "I'm from Huntsville. I'm a student," Taylor told him.

King asked him if he'd eaten yet and whether he had a place to stay for the night. Taylor told him that he and the others had brought sandwiches and that they planned to return to Huntsville after the trial. And then King shook his hand. "If I had known it was so important, I never would have washed that hand again, you see," Taylor said.

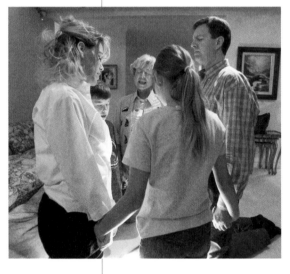

An Adventist family gathers for prayer in their home.

I'm sure Taylor has told that story hundreds of times before. But it had a special meaning for me because of a conversation we were having about longevity. Taylor had told me a few other things about his life, including episodes of racial discrimination, and I'd asked him if he'd like to live longer. Did he have a goal to reach a certain age?

"Not really," he replied. As a man of faith, he had no fear of death.

But if that was true, I asked, then why bother eating well, getting exercise, observing the Sabbath, and doing all the other things that the Adventists have shown will extend your years?

"I just don't do this so that I won't die," he said. "When you have a relationship with Jesus Christ, you are at peace." He recalled what King had said in Memphis on the night before he was assassinated: *I've been to the mountaintop.* "In the language and the culture of the Black church, that means you can see what God has for you," Taylor said. "You don't have a fear of death."

"And that's the philosophy that Adventism has helped you to embrace?"

He nodded and launched into another story about Ellen White and her

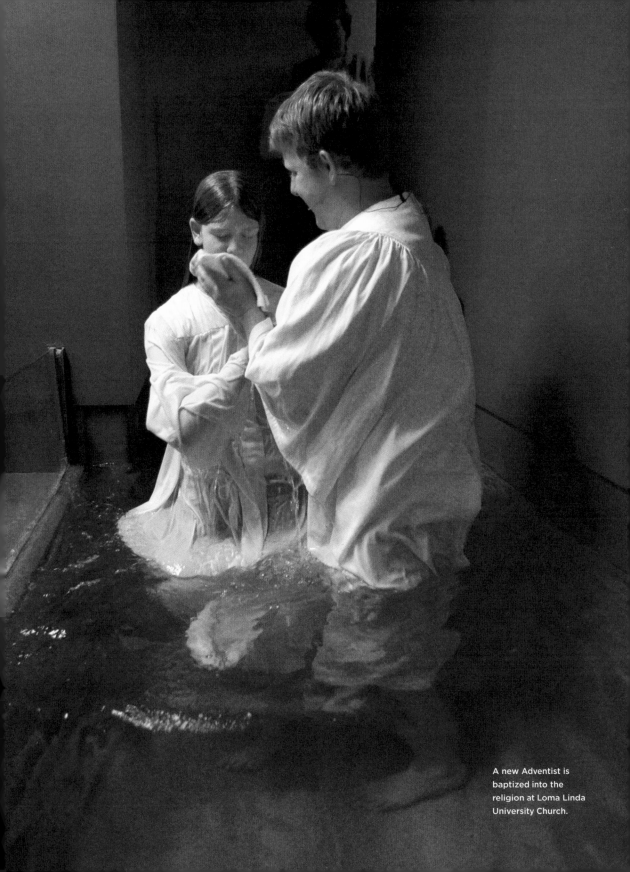

A new Adventist is baptized into the religion at Loma Linda University Church.

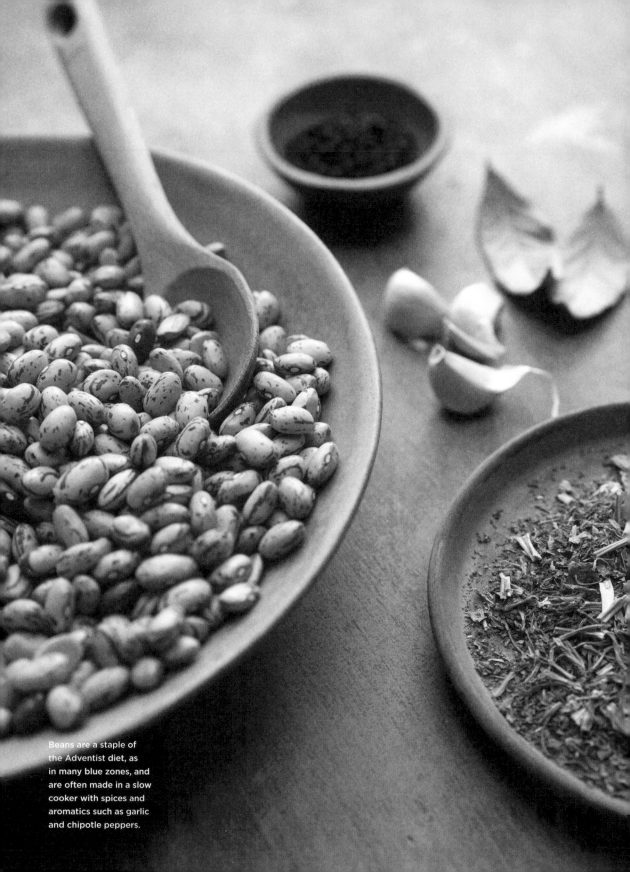

Beans are a staple of the Adventist diet, as in many blue zones, and are often made in a slow cooker with spices and aromatics such as garlic and chipotle peppers.

# Top Longevity Foods From Loma Linda

M ore than half of the foods in the Adventist diet come from fruits and vegetables. A study at Loma Linda University confirms that strict vegetarian Adventists can expect to live nearly a decade longer than other Americans, while suffering fewer chronic diseases and cancers. Their plant-based diet was strongly influenced by Ellen G. White, one of the 19th-century founders of the Adventist church, who wrote that "grains, fruits, nuts, and vegetables constitute the diet chosen for us by our Creator. These foods, prepared in as simple and natural a manner as possible, are the most healthful and nourishing."

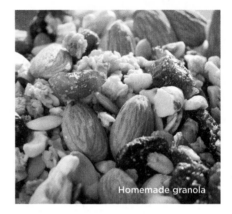
Homemade granola

**SOY MILK** | High in protein and low in fat, soy milk—not the sweetened, flavored kind—is used as an alternative to dairy. It contains phytoestrogens that may protect against some types of cancer.

**WEETABIX** | A whole-grain cereal mostly sold in England, Weetabix adds whole grains to Loma Linda diets. It also promotes skin and bone health and keeps you regular, among other benefits.

**CORNFLAKES** | A staple of the Adventist breakfast, cornflakes are rich in vitamins and minerals like folate and thiamine.

**BREWER'S YEAST** | This dietary supplement contains chromium, which may help control blood sugar levels and improve glucose tolerance. It also has immune-boosting properties.

**NUTS** | A key part of Adventist diets, nuts and nut butters have been found to add two to three years to lifespans when a handful are eaten at least five times a week.

**OATMEAL** | A staple for Adventists, slow-cooked oatmeal provides a balanced portion of fats, complex carbohydrates, and plant protein, along with a good dose of iron and B vitamins.

**AVOCADOS** | High in potassium and low in salt, avocados may help reduce blood pressure and the risk of stroke. Ounce for ounce, an avocado contains 30 percent more potassium than a banana.

**VEGEMITE** | Made from brewer's yeast, salt, and vegetable extract, this Australian spread is perfect for topping whole wheat toast and an excellent source of vitamins that support brain health.

**BEANS** | As in all blue zones, beans are king. For the vegetarian Adventists, beans, lentils, and peas represent an important daily protein source.

**SPINACH** | Green vegetables such as spinach and broccoli provide essential vitamins, minerals, and fiber.

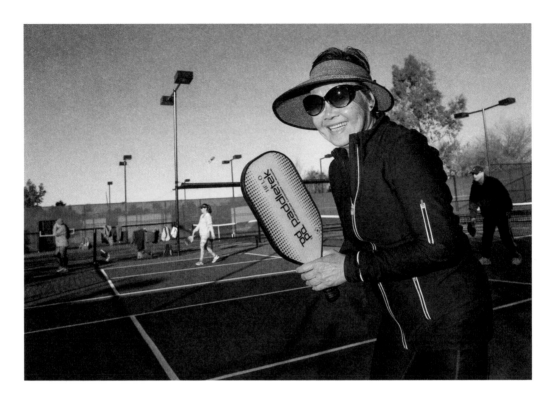

Lee Maxwell, 66, plays pickleball during a senior activities class at Loma Linda University's Drayson Center.

life, and it struck me how powerfully the Adventist faith supports its adherents. Even when faced with a lifetime of challenges, including racial prejudice, Taylor had the strength to stay on the path.

No wonder then, that Adventists have been so successful at resisting life's many other temptations, whether it's smoking, eating cheeseburgers, or spending the weekend on the couch binge-watching TV. They're doubly motivated to eat a whole-food, plant-based diet because it's both healthy and holy. They know it's better for them, but they also believe their bodies are a temple of the Lord, which they must keep clean and strong.

Adventists also find purpose in their relationship with Jesus, which provides them with a clear path in life. They find refreshment in their observation of the Sabbath, which recharges their batteries with friendships, family time, and fresh air. They volunteer, which gets older people out of the house and nourishes their sense of meaning. And they hang out with other Adventists, which reinforces all their other healthy behaviors, whether they're playing pickleball or going to Zumba class or sharing food at a potluck.

"So, how much of your health and vitality and sharpness of mind do you attribute to your faith and your belief in God?" I asked Taylor. "And how much of it is your willful effort to eat right and sleep and get exercise and so on?"

Instead of answering, he told me another story.

During a recent visit to his personal doctor, he'd noticed an odd expression creep onto the physician's face.

"What's wrong?" Taylor had asked.

The doctor had smiled. "Did you know that you've grown a quarter of an inch taller?"

Taylor was surprised. "Then I got very theological on him," he said. He told his doctor that when people got to be his age, they often bent over, looking for a hole in the ground. "But as an Adventist, one who loves the Lord, I'm looking for the hole in the sky."

Taylor laughed as he finished the story.

"You should be a preacher," I said.

The church kitchen is busy during one of the many potlucks that bring Adventists together after worshipping.

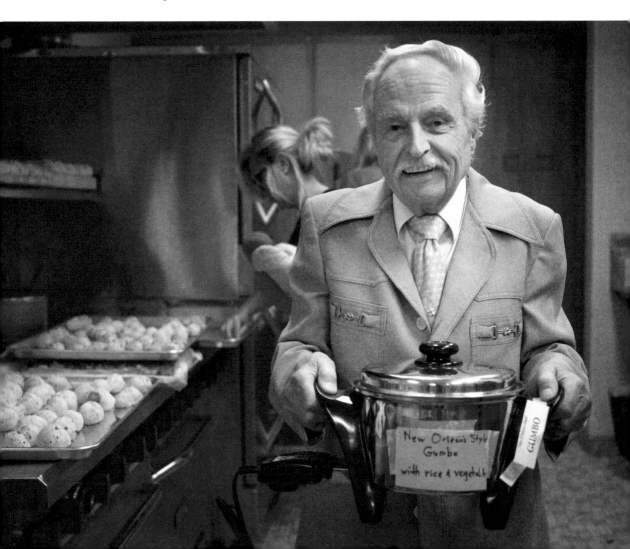

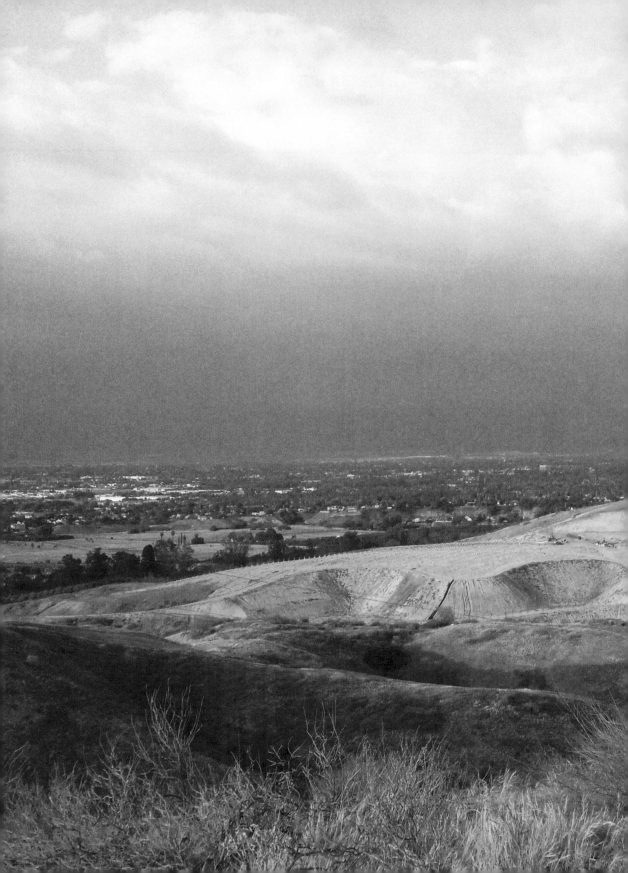

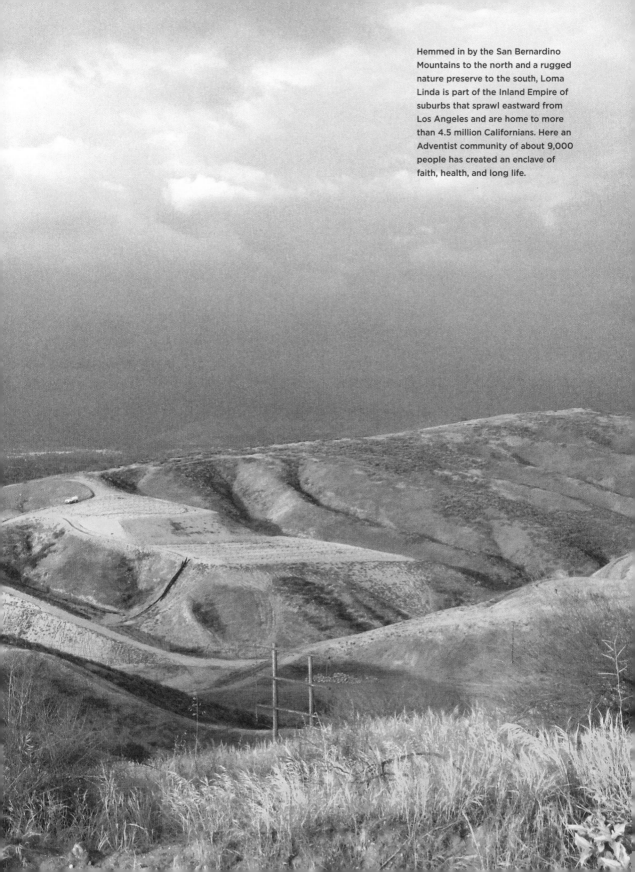

Hemmed in by the San Bernardino Mountains to the north and a rugged nature preserve to the south, Loma Linda is part of the Inland Empire of suburbs that sprawl eastward from Los Angeles and are home to more than 4.5 million Californians. Here an Adventist community of about 9,000 people has created an enclave of faith, health, and long life.

# LESSONS FROM LOMA LINDA'S BLUE ZONE

■ **Find a sanctuary in time**

The 24-hour Sabbath provides a time to focus on family, God, camaraderie, and nature. Adventists claim this relieves their stress, strengthens social networks, and provides consistent exercise.

■ **Watch your body mass index (BMI)**

Adventists have healthier BMIs than the average American. Studies correlate excess weight with a higher risk of heart attack, stroke, high blood pressure, diabetes, arthritis, and several cancers.

■ **Get regular, moderate exercise**

The Adventist Health Studies show that getting regular, low-intensity exercise—like taking daily walks—appears to reduce chances of heart disease and cancers.

■ **Spend time with like-minded friends**

Adventists tend to spend time with lots of other Adventists. They find well-being by sharing one another's values and supporting one another's beliefs.

■ **Snack on nuts**

Adventists who consume nuts at least five times a week have about half the risk of heart disease and live about two years longer than those who don't. At least four major studies have confirmed that eating nuts has a positive impact on health and life expectancy.

■ **Give something back**

Adventism, like many faiths, encourages and provides opportunities for volunteerism. Often the centenarians we spoke with stay active, find a sense of purpose, and stave off depression by focusing on helping others.

■ **Avoid meat**

Many Adventists follow a vegetarian or vegan diet. The AHS studies show that consuming fruits, vegetables, and whole grains seems to be protective against a wide variety of cancers. The longest-lived Adventists are vegetarian or pescatarian.

■ **Eat an early light dinner**

"Eat breakfast like a king, lunch like a prince, and dinner like a pauper," American nutritionist Adelle Davis is said to have recommended—an attitude also reflected in Adventist practices. A light dinner early in the evening avoids flooding the body with calories during the inactive parts of the day. It also seems to promote better sleep and a lower BMI.

■ **Drink plenty of water**

The AHS studies suggest that men who drank five or six daily glasses of water had a substantial reduction in the risk of a fatal heart attack—by 60 to 70 percent—compared with those who drank considerably less.

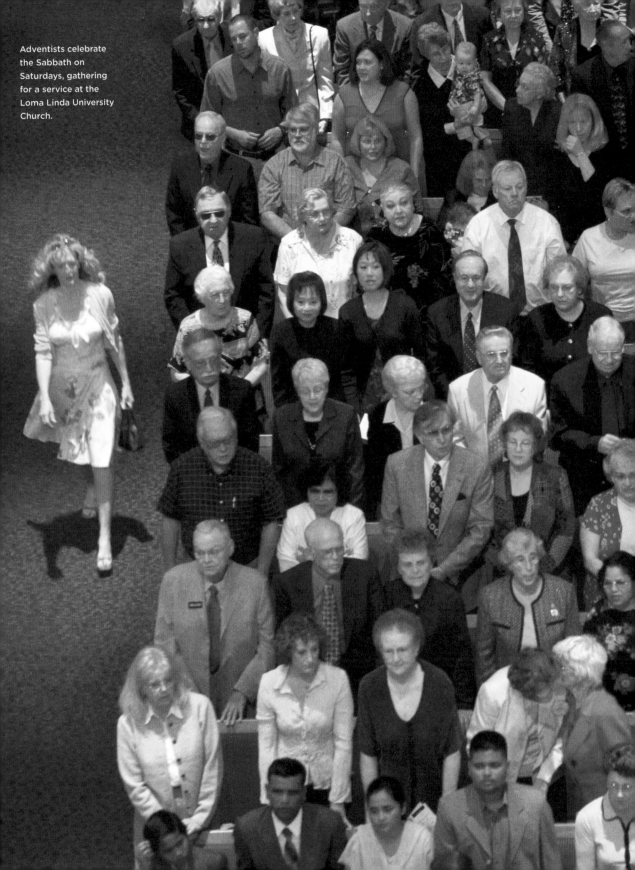

Adventists celebrate the Sabbath on Saturdays, gathering for a service at the Loma Linda University Church.

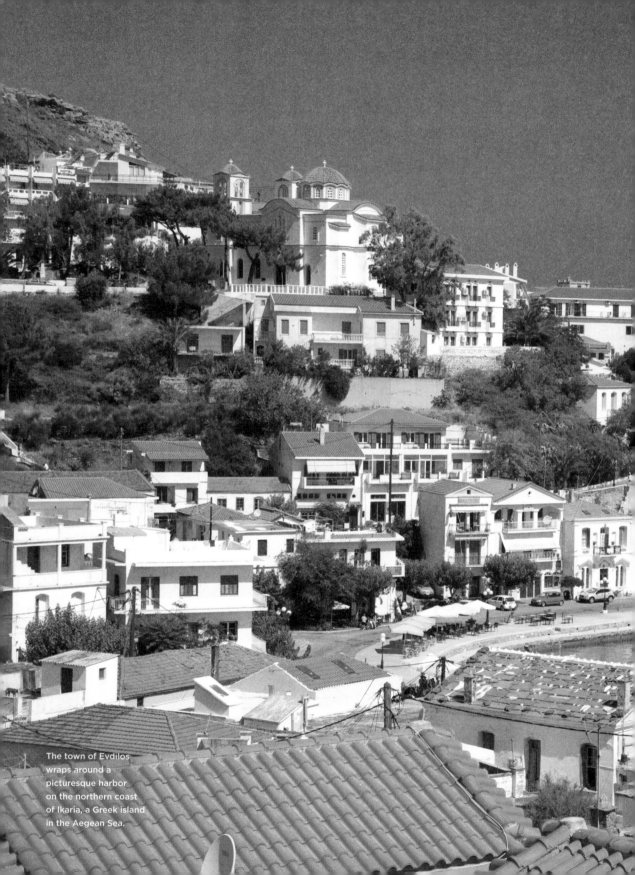

The town of Evdilos wraps around a picturesque harbor on the northern coast of Ikaria, a Greek island in the Aegean Sea.

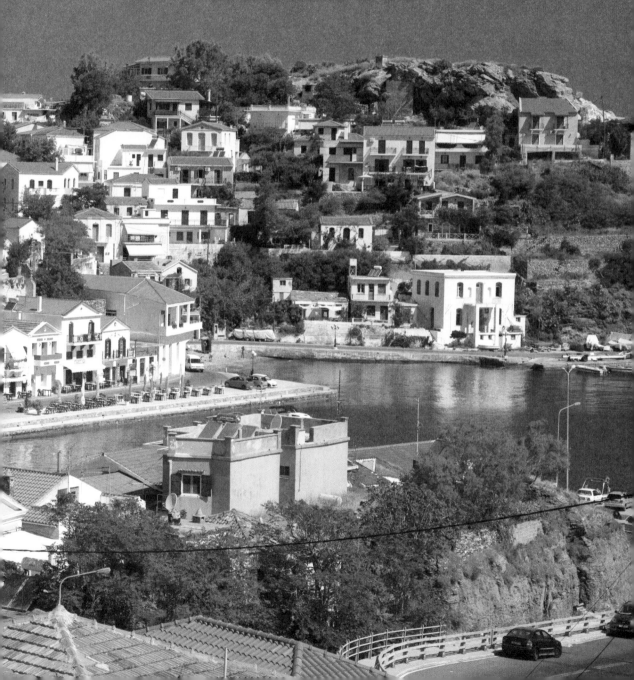

CHAPTER 4

# Ikaria

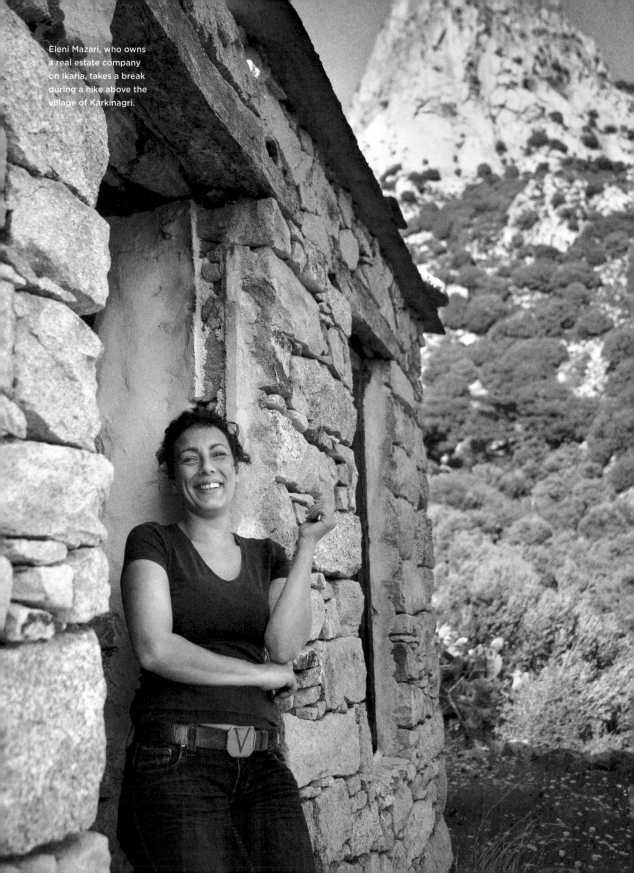

Eleni Mazari, who owns a real estate company on Ikaria, takes a break during a hike above the village of Karkinagri.

# Where People "Forget to Die"

The inscrutable island of Ikaria resembles a half-submerged *Brontosaurus* that has waded across the eastern Aegean Sea from the coast of Turkey and stretched out for a nap. Here, in isolated homesteads above steeply terraced gardens and vineyards, you'll find yet another remarkable group of long-lived people—Greek nationals who live an average of eight years longer than most Americans, with half the rate of our heart disease and barely a fifth the rate of our dementia.

Isolated by time, tradition, and rampaging winds, the 10,000 inhabitants of this small island have fashioned a unique culture—one that promotes a healthy diet of wild greens, beans, olive oil, sourdough bread, and strong red wine, along with late-night games of dominoes and a relaxed pace of life that pays little attention to clocks.

Like most of the other blue zones, Ikaria is remote, and its residents have stuck to time-honored traditions that have helped them get through hard times and avoid harmful modern influences. Junk food is all but unknown here, and the people don't stumble through their days glued to their phones. Instead, clean air, warm breezes, and a rugged terrain draw them outdoors to pursue active lifestyles that help one in three make it into their nineties.

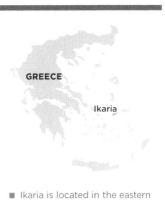

**GREECE**

Ikaria

- Ikaria is located in the eastern part of the Aegean Sea near Turkey.

- The islanders eat a version of the Mediterranean diet.

- One in three residents makes it to their 90s.

- Ikarians suffer half the rate of heart disease that Americans do.

Unlike in other blue zones, residents of the island tend to live in small, isolated homesteads rather than clustering in villages. Although there are three main population centers—Christos Raches, Evdilos, and Agios Kirykos—most of the people live out on the land. This pattern, established centuries ago, enables each family to be relatively self-sufficient, with enough property for a garden, an orchard, and maybe a vineyard. Work in the fields goes late into the day, prompting shops in the nearby small towns to remain closed until the evening hours. People stay up late, especially in the summer, and older folks take naps, which has been associated with a one-third lower rate of heart disease.

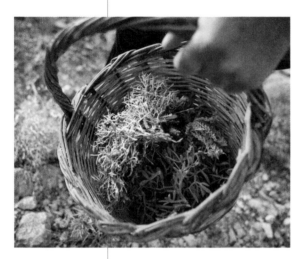

Many varieties of herbs grow wild on the rugged slopes.

This simple way of life and the extraordinary longevity of Ikarians were both noted centuries ago by Joseph Georgirenes, the archbishop of Samos and Ikaria. As he wrote in 1677, "The most commendable thing of this Island is their Air and Water, both so healthful, that the People are very long liv'd, it being an ordinary thing to see persons in it of an 100 years of Age, which is a great wonder, considering how hardily they live."

Describing Ikaria as "Mountainous and full of Rocks," he noted that it had "a great many little Villages scattered up and down through the whole Island." The people were so poor, he wrote, neither the Turks nor the barbarous pirates considered them worth bothering. Their food and clothing were worse than that of beggars in other countries. And yet, he concluded, the people on Ikaria were the happiest in the Aegean. "The Soil is Barren, but the Air is Healthful; their Wealth is but small, but their Liberty and Security is great."

In keeping with this tradition of austerity—unemployment has been as high as 40 percent in recent years—Ikarians still harvest much of their food from their own land or gather it from the wild. Besides eating vegetables from their gardens, islanders also consume dozens of different greens that grow in the nearby hills. During my visits to the island, I often see women by the side of a road with a knife in one hand and a sack in the other brimming with fennel fronds, parsley, samphire, wild dandelions, or chicory. Most of the plants they collect look like something an American would hit with a Weedwacker. And yet, as I noted in my book *The Blue Zones Kitchen,* these rich greens contain a bounty in antioxidants—10 times as many as red wine—and make for tasty dishes when boiled and baked into pies or added to salads.

Ikaria's relative isolation has also encouraged an outsize camaraderie among its people. Their allegiance is to family first and then to other islanders in a spirit of mutual care. (Greece comes in a distant third in terms of loyalty.) Instead of sitting on the couch watching TV, people get together with family and friends on a regular basis, and they look after one another.

This is especially true of the oldest Ikarians. Romain Legrand, from Dijon University Hospital, and a team of French researchers recently reported that among Ikarians in their nineties, more than three-quarters engage in social contacts with neighbors, friends, or family every day. "In the villages, the participants would often meet with friends at the 'kafenio' or continue an activity in one of the village stores," they wrote in a 2021 study. Such social connections provided "beneficial effects on health, improving the prognosis of cardiovascular and neurovascular diseases, such as myocardial infarction and stroke, reducing mortality risk, and improving mental health."

Villagers drape their arms over one another's shoulders as they dance the Ikariotikos at an annual *panigiri* festival.

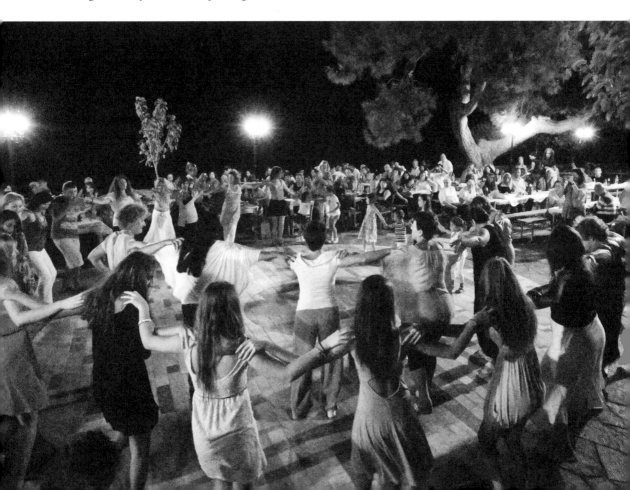

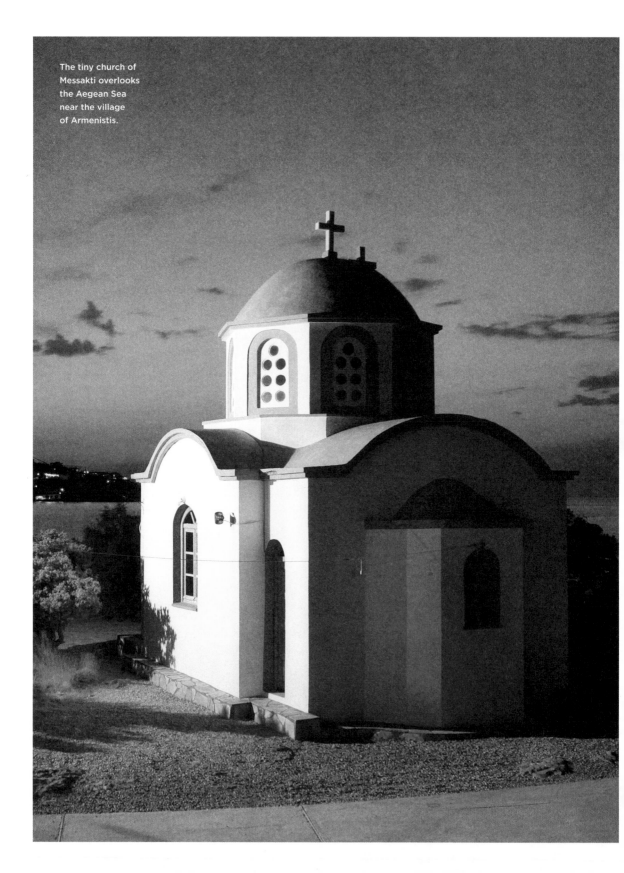

The tiny church of Messakti overlooks the Aegean Sea near the village of Armenistis.

No one had to explain the benefits of love and friendship to Aleka and Paniote Mazari, who recently welcomed me to their snug little house surrounded by olive trees, a garden, and a vineyard. Their kitchen was clean and compact, with knickknacks on the shelf above an open fireplace. Aleka, 85, had baked a beautiful cake for my visit, as well as a plate of cookies. She wore her blond hair up in a messy bun. A brown scarf was coiled around her neck, and she moved around the kitchen with energy.

"How do you maintain your vigor?" I asked when she finally sat down.

Paniote, 97, put his arm around his wife and kissed her. "I show you," he said.

She laughed as he pawed at her.

Paniote was wearing a blue-green cardigan. "I wouldn't be here if it weren't for her," he said. "She gives me all of her care, and the love, and the sweet life."

The two met late in life, they said. They'd both been married before. But Paniote remembered having seen Aleka at the beach many years earlier—the same beach where she'd swum her whole life and still swims today. After the death of his wife, Paniote spotted her again at a gathering. When she walked in, it was like an electric shock, he said. He worked up the courage to speak to her, which she said prompted "a tickle in my soul." Aleka was 57; Paniote was 69.

Studies have shown that climbing hills every day contributes to the long lives of shepherds.

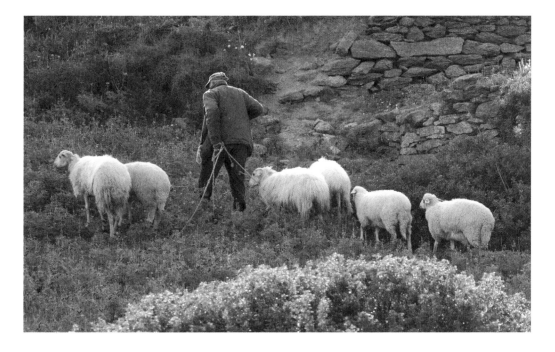

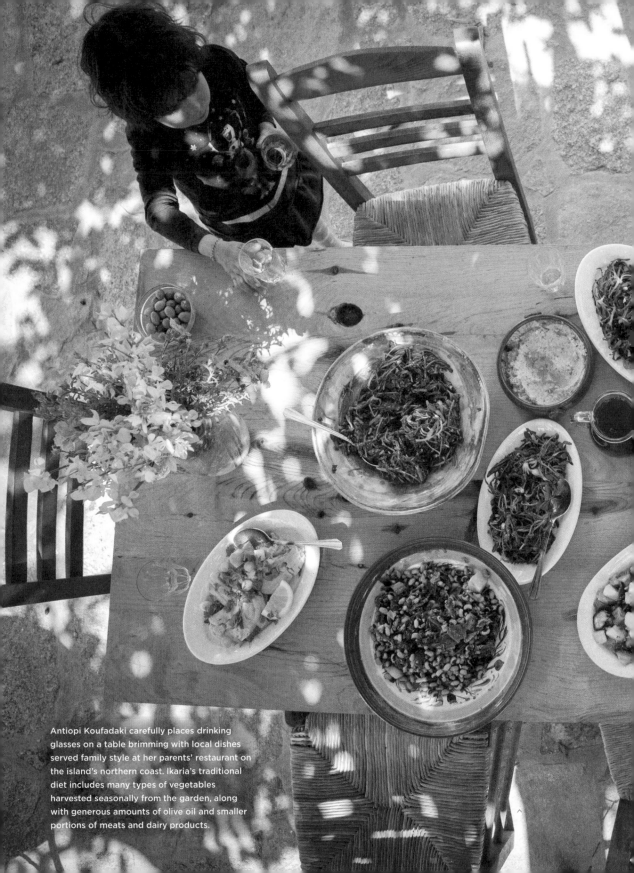

Antiopi Koufadaki carefully places drinking glasses on a table brimming with local dishes served family style at her parents' restaurant on the island's northern coast. Ikaria's traditional diet includes many types of vegetables harvested seasonally from the garden, along with generous amounts of olive oil and smaller portions of meats and dairy products.

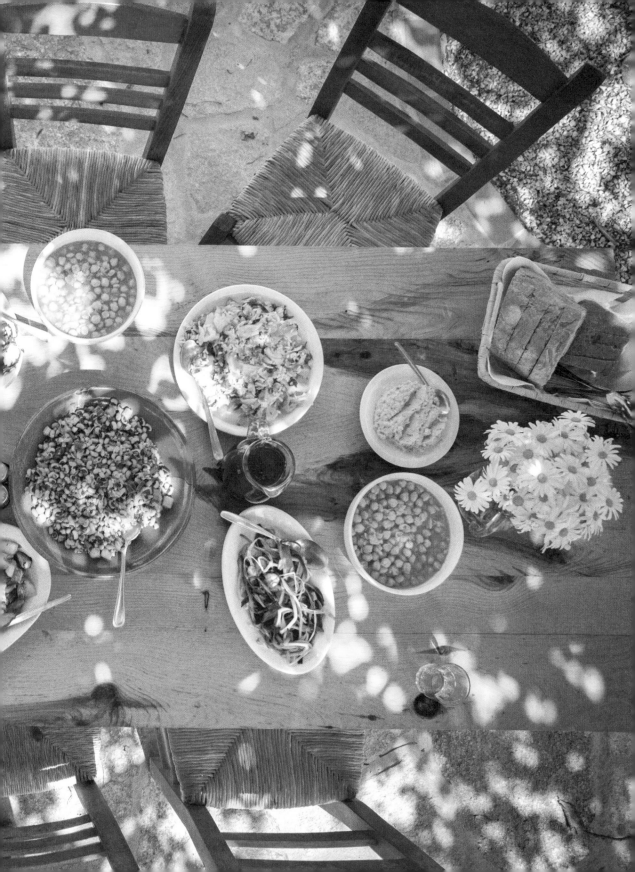

Still, it took him more than a month to convince her to go out with him. "She was a tough walnut," he said. They dated secretly at first. He'd pick her up in his truck, and they'd hide from the rest of the village. But eventually his children found out. They got married seven years later. And now, despite their advanced years, they say they're still the ones at the party who get everyone else up to dance.

"She brought me back to life," Paniote said.

The science backs him up. Being married has been shown to help you live longer, with greater happiness. In the recent French study, most of the Ikarian men in their nineties were married, which the researchers speculated might also help explain the curious lack of depression on the island.

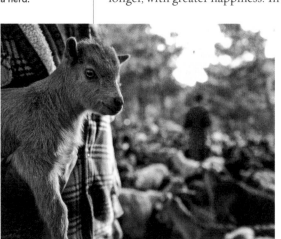

Staying active helps, too. Like Aleka Mazari, 80 percent of the seniors interviewed by the French team still swam in the Aegean past their 75th year. Nearly three-fourths reported they kept active with moderate to high physical activity, such as working in the family vineyard or walking up and down the steep hills to church or the village. Such activities have been known to reduce the risks of diseases ranging from cardiovascular illness to diabetes, cancer, and depression. "Of particular importance to older adults, physical activity reduces risk and injury from falls, and prevents or delays cognitive impairment and disability," the researchers wrote.

Both of these ingredients for good health—social connections and staying active—come together every summer at Ikaria's famous village festivals, called *panigíria*. Originally held to celebrate the name days of Christian Orthodox saints, these community-building celebrations invite islanders of all ages to eat, drink, and link arms as they dance the Ikariotikos.

More than 90 panigiria take place on Ikaria from May to September. I attended a joyous one a few years ago in the village of Lefkada, where the men roasted goats and the women served salads of various kinds with copious wine from local vineyards. The small price of admission went toward a community project.

The party went on all night, as I recall, and what impressed me most was

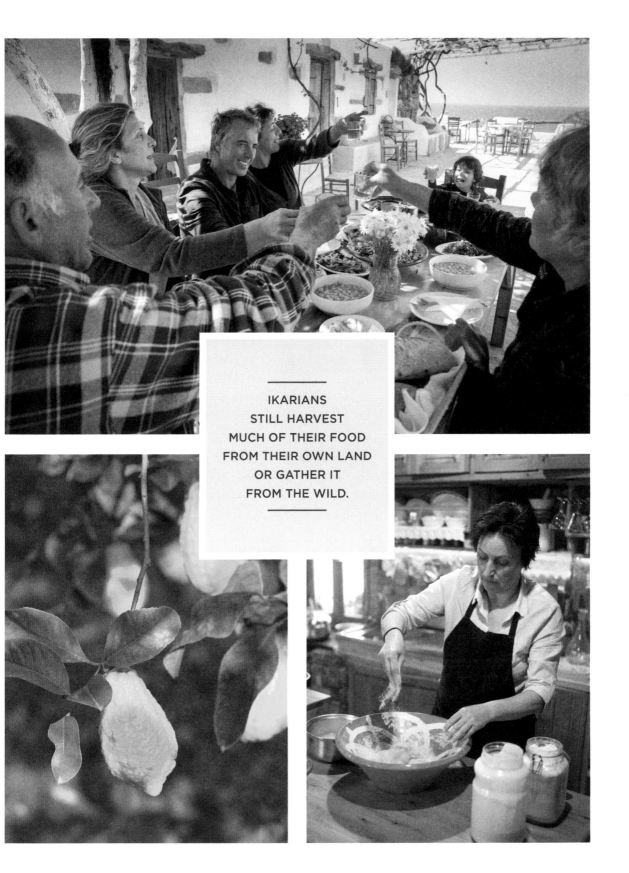

IKARIANS
STILL HARVEST
MUCH OF THEIR FOOD
FROM THEIR OWN LAND
OR GATHER IT
FROM THE WILD.

that everyone participated, from eight-year-olds to eighty-year-olds. Men and women were up on their feet, draping their arms over their neighbors' shoulders, and dancing in mesmerizing circles, sort of sashaying and gently kicking, until everyone was misty eyed with a blend of community, family, and island pride.

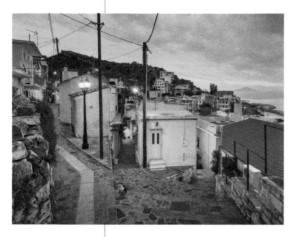

In a positive sign for Ikaria, the younger generation has lately shown an interest in preserving, or bringing back, such traditions. This is almost unique among the world's blue zones, where the old ways are steadily being replaced by modern habits.

"We were brought up to love Ikaria," said Philipo Karimalis, a 47-year-old lawyer. "But in the 1980s and 1990s, the rustic life became uncool. Young people didn't want to go to panigiria anymore. Then in the 2000s they started going again. The festivals sparked a reinterest in the traditional ways."

*Agios Kirykos, where a sunset lights up the sky*

As we sat together on his patio, he poured me some of his homemade wine made from an ancient variety of grape he'd discovered in his grandfather's vineyard. The wine was fermented in amphorae, rather than barrels, and sealed with local beeswax. We enjoyed the wine with sourdough bread, homemade cheese, and a Greek salad with mint.

I asked him if foods like these might be part of the recipe for Ikaria's longevity.

"Of course," he said. "Ikarians are made of wine, honey, and olive oil.

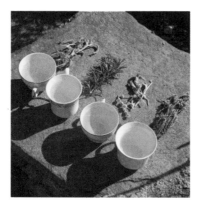

## HERBAL TEAS

Many Ikarians treat themselves to a cup of herbal tea every day, often using wild herbs harvested from the rocky island and sweetened with local honey. Poppy tea is considered a mild relaxant, while chicory tea provides energy, rosemary tea enhances skin and digestion, and thyme tea is taken for allergy relief and coughs. Sage teas are thought to treat colds and even act as a natural Viagra, while mountain tea (made from Sideritis plants) is good for flu, headaches, and colds. Many common herbs act as mild diuretics and contain antioxidants and anti-inflammatory properties, which may contribute to Ikaria's low rates of cardiovascular disease and dementia.

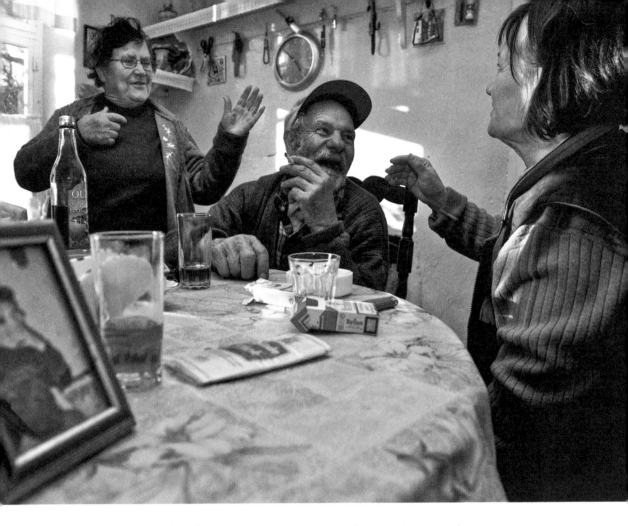

A centenarian shares a laugh with his sisters over a drink and a smoke.

Growing your own garden, fermenting your own wine, and supporting your neighbors—these are what keep people here living longer."

Dr. Christina Chrysohoou tends to agree. The cardiologist from the University of Athens Medical School was among the first academics to study Ikaria's diet and health habits. In 2009 she and Demosthenes B. Panagiotakos of Harokopio University organized the Ikaria Study, surveying 1,410 Ikarians, including 79 over the age of 90, which was a significantly higher number than you would expect based on the European average.

She and her research team confirmed that Ikarians had adopted an extreme and unique version of the Mediterranean diet, which included vegetables, whole grains, fruits, fish, olive oil, goat's milk and cheese, and wine. What set the islanders apart was that they consumed less fish than others in the region but showed a heftier appetite for potatoes, beans and legumes such as chickpeas, lentils, and black-eyed peas, and for wild greens such as dandelion, chicory,

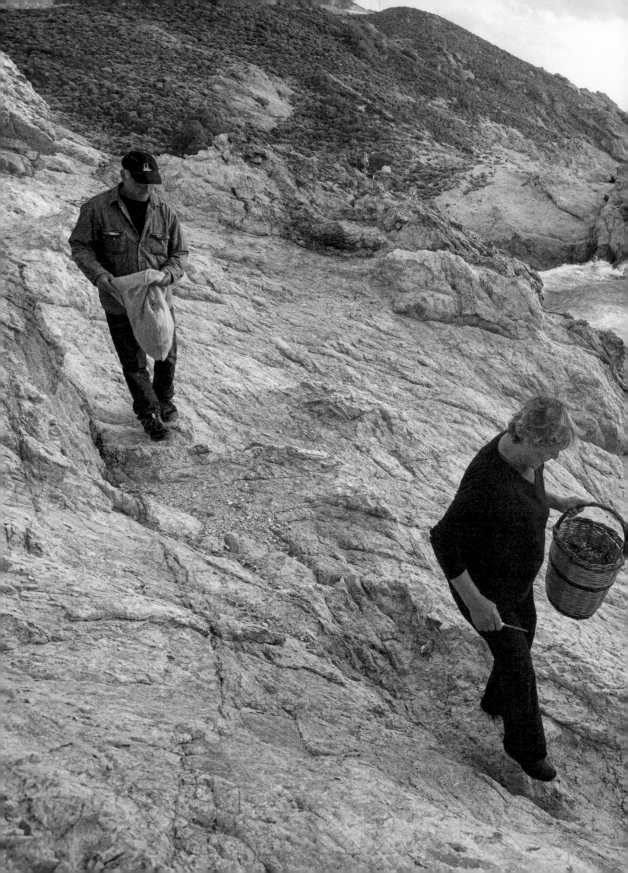

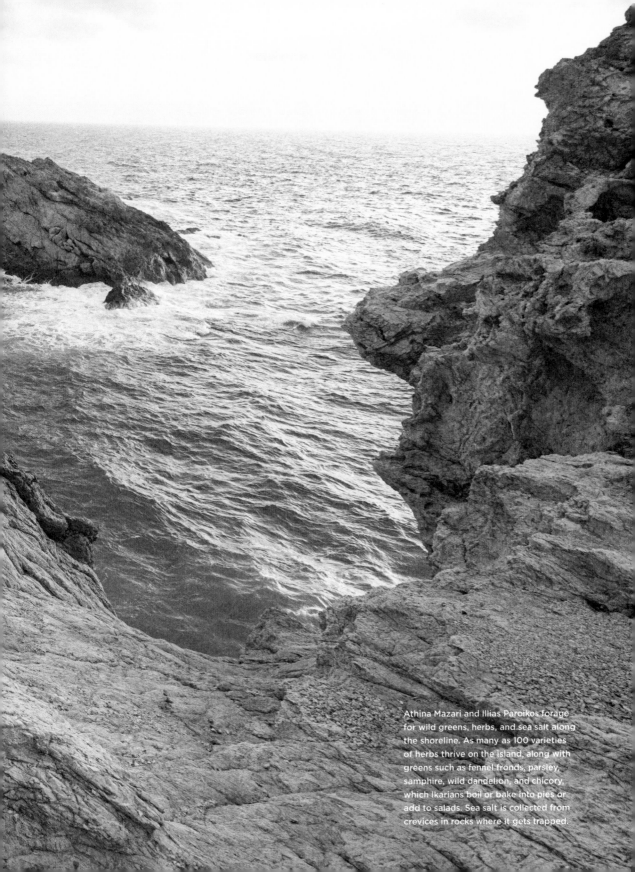

Athina Mazari and Illias Paroikos forage for wild greens, herbs, and sea salt along the shoreline. As many as 100 varieties of herbs thrive on the island, along with greens such as fennel fronds, parsley, samphire, wild dandelion, and chicory, which Ikarians boil or bake into pies or add to salads. Sea salt is collected from crevices in rocks where it gets trapped.

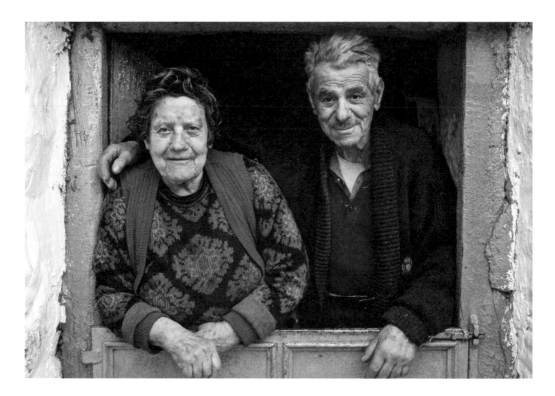

Vlasis Giakis, 98, and his wife, Eleytheria, pose in their doorway. A recent study has shown that most Ikarian men in their 90s are married.

and wild fennel, which they dried on roofs or hung in mesh bags for storage if they had extra.

But the Ikaria study went further. Besides highlighting the islanders' healthy diet, it also pointed out that older Ikarians kept active both physically and socially, took regular naps, and continued to have sex. As other research has shown, taking a 30-minute nap at least five times a week can lower stress hormones and reduce your risk of heart attack by more than a third. Even though more than a fourth of those in the study still smoked, Ikarians as a whole managed to live about eight years longer than people elsewhere while avoiding heart disease, diabetes, stroke, and dementia. In fact, as Chrysohoou and her colleagues reported, 90-year-olds on Ikaria suffered no more disease, on average, than most people in their sixties.

We learned more about the health effects of Ikarian foods from Ioanna Chinou of Athens University, a leading authority on the bioactive properties of herbs. People on the island sip herbal teas all day, whether they're made with oregano, mint, rosemary, marjoram, or some other plant from the garden or the field. During one of my earlier trips to Ikaria, I sent samples of these herbal teas to Chinou to be laboratory-tested. She reported that they all had

# Chickpea Soup
# With Lemon and Herbs

TOTAL COOK TIME: 2 HOURS, 20 MINUTES; 45 MINUTES IF USING CANNED CHICKPEAS • SERVES 6

Greeks, and Ikarians especially, have mastered the blend of lemon, olive oil, and herbs. This simple soup is a warming alternative to chicken soup in the winter, and yet another way to creatively make beans taste good and figure into your daily diet. Chickpea soup is one of the most classic comfort foods in Ikaria and even throughout the rest of Greece—you'll find it in almost every home and tavern.

1 pound dried chickpeas, soaked overnight, rinsed, and peeled (or four 15-ounce cans low-sodium chickpeas, drained)

1 medium onion, coarsely chopped

1 garlic clove, minced

1 bay leaf

½ cup extra-virgin olive oil, plus more for serving

Salt and pepper

Juice of 3 lemons, for serving

Place the drained chickpeas in a pot with just enough water to cover, and bring them to a boil. Remove from the heat, drain, rinse, and put them into a clean pot.

Add the onion, garlic, bay leaf, olive oil, and enough water to cover the ingredients. Stir to combine.

If using dried chickpeas, bring to a boil and then simmer for about 2 hours, or until chickpeas are soft.

If using canned chickpeas, bring to a boil and then simmer for 30 minutes, adding a few tablespoons of water at a time to thin the soup as needed.

Remove from the heat and discard the bay leaf. Add salt and pepper to taste.

Serve with generous drizzles of lemon juice and olive oil.

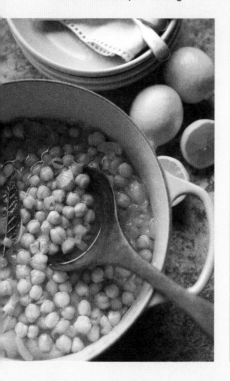

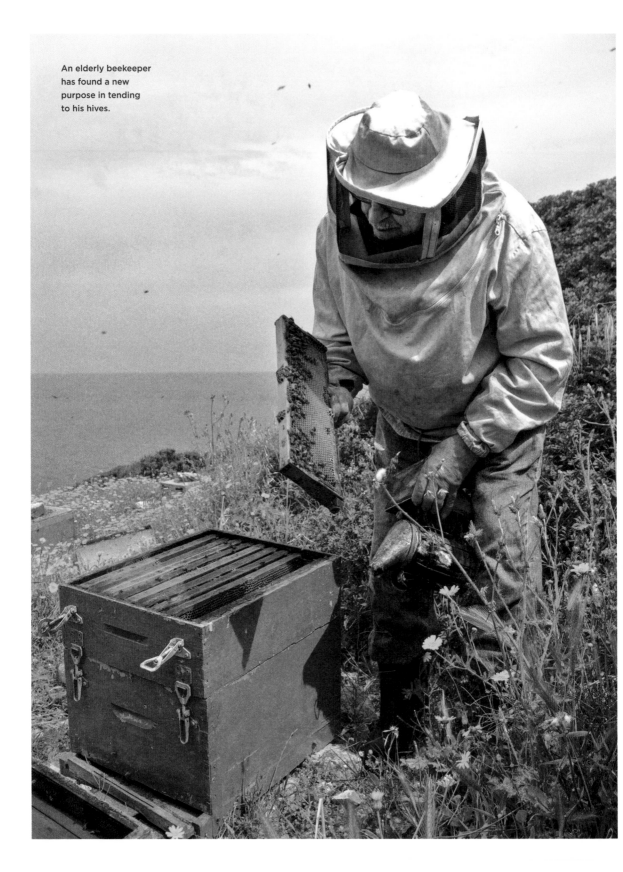

An elderly beekeeper has found a new purpose in tending to his hives.

antioxidant properties in addition to functioning as mild diuretics. Not only did they contain powerful antioxidants, in other words; they might also help flush waste products from the body and slightly lower blood pressure. When added to cooked dishes, fresh herbs offer similar health benefits.

So much for the science behind the Ikarian lifestyle. Near the end of a recent visit to the island, I returned to the home of an old friend whose story, more than any other I've encountered, captured the mystery of the place.

His name was Stamatis Moraitis, and when he was still in his mid-sixties, living and working in the United States, he was diagnosed with lung cancer. His doctors gave him six to nine months to live. Resigned to his fate, he moved back to his native Ikaria with his wife, Elpiniki, and moved in with his elderly parents near Evdilos, intending to be buried with his ancestors in a shady cemetery overlooking the Aegean.

The months came and went while he cleaned up his parents' vineyard and worked in their garden. Without really thinking about it, he eased into the rhythms of Ikarian life, taking an afternoon nap and later strolling down to the local tavern to play dominoes. He fixed up his parents' house and made wine from their grapes. And his cancer seemingly disappeared. Three and a half decades later, when I met up with him in 2012, he was still going strong at 97.

Four generations: Eleni Mazari enjoys a meal with her daughter Antiopi, mother Athina, and grandmother Katerina Karoutsou.

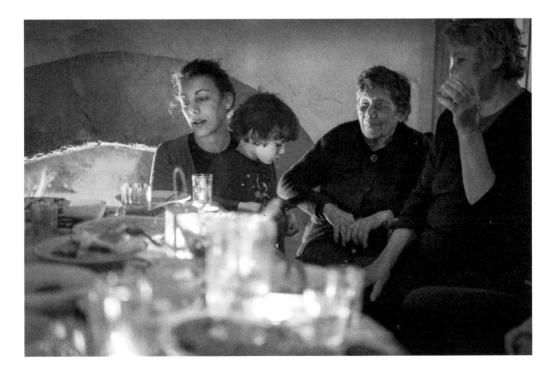

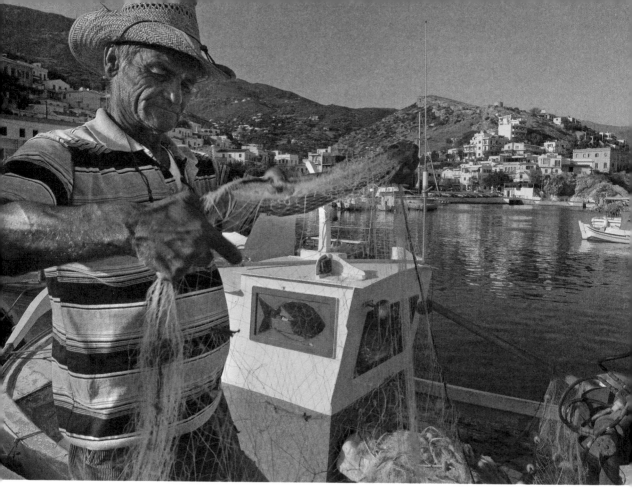

Moraitis died soon thereafter, still cancer free. He'd never undergone chemotherapy nor been treated in any way for his disease. All he'd done was return to Ikaria.

I stopped by his small whitewashed house this past spring. The place looked abandoned, with bushes growing up in his olive grove and weeds taking over his vineyard. I recalled strolling through these same fruit trees with him, picking ripe oranges and lemons as he told his favorite stories. Moraitis was short and nearly bald, except for a few rebellious strands that furtively covered his scalp, and he always had a mischievous grin on his lips.

His grandson, Christoforos Yeralis, let me into the house. He wore jeans, sneakers, and a T-shirt with necklaces, and he looked shockingly like Moraitis, except for his full head of hair. He had his grandfather's sense of humor, too, and he told me what a partygoer Moraitis had been, careening around the island's curvy roads in his aging Lada station wagon.

The house had been packed up, more or less, pictures taken off the walls.

All except for Moraitis's bedroom, which was still intact. We found a small chest Yeralis hadn't noticed before and opened it with a key. Inside was a treasure trove of old photos, showing Moraitis and various members of his family. Yeralis remembered going fishing with his grandfather and helping him with his little olive grove and vineyard.

We opened the windows and the golden afternoon light poured in. I had expected to feel melancholic returning to Moraitis's house this way. But surprisingly, I didn't. He'd lived a full life for almost a century, 63 years with a loving wife, and he'd found happiness on the island, working in his orchard and vineyard and with his olives. In the end, he'd been buried in his ancestral graveyard, just as he'd hoped.

A toast to good health from Giannis Karimalis, 78, who was diagnosed with cancer four decades earlier

I found the cemetery at the end of a dirt road, perched on a terrace on the side of a cliff, shaded by cedar trees, with an unbelievable view of the Aegean. The sun sets every day on his tombstone, where someone had put a picture of him in a glass case. I smiled to see Moraitis again in his poorly matched blue plaid shirt and brown plaid shorts, a mischievous grin on his face.

I thought of something my friend Gianni Pes, the University of Sassari medical statistician, had once said about the Ikarian way of dying. Pes had analyzed the best data on the island's extraordinary longevity and reached a very Ikarian conclusion. People on the island manage for a long time to avoid the diseases that kill most other people, he said. "But eventually they still have to die. So they are dying in the Ikarian way—they take time. And, by doing so, they live longer."

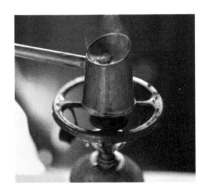

## IKARIAN COFFEE

A daily ritual for many islanders, Ikarian coffee is served foamy and rich to friends and family gathered in cafés. Brewed in a small pot called a *briki,* the coffee is prepared using a process similar to that found in Turkey and the Middle East. Boiling the grounds and waiting for them to settle to the bottom is thought to release healthful compounds from the beans, along with protective antioxidants and polyphenols. The resulting coffee also delivers less caffeine than you would normally get in a typical cup of American coffee, reducing the chances of unwelcome side effects from the caffeine.

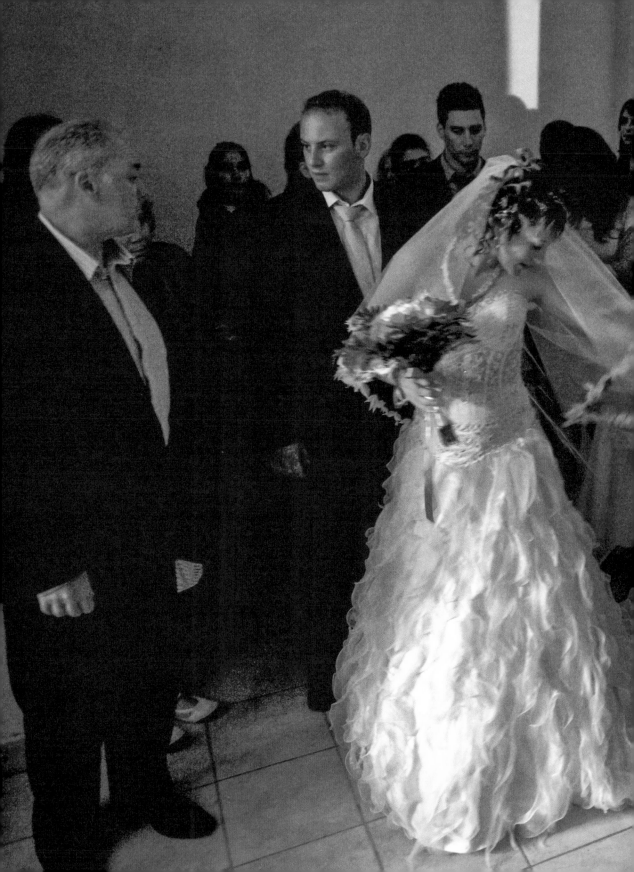

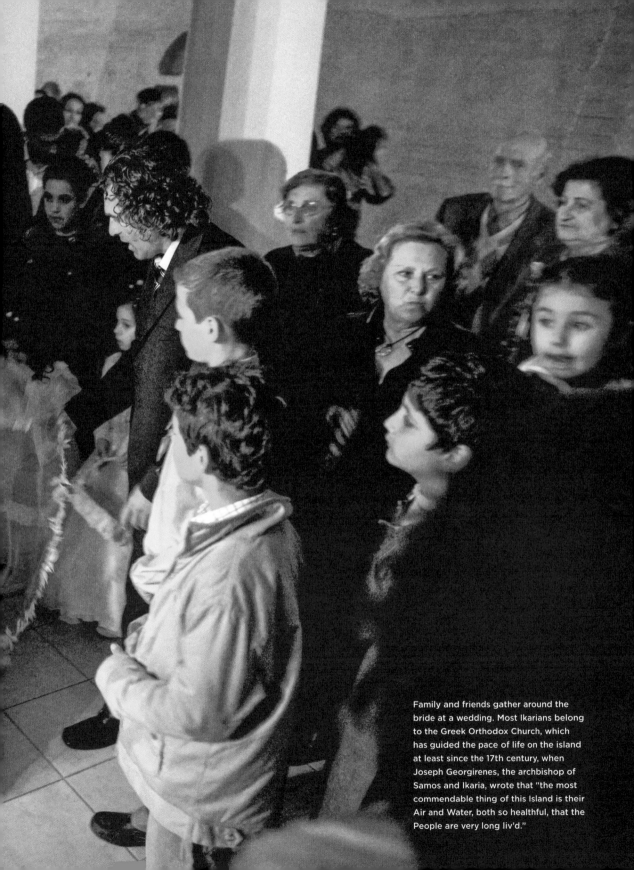

Family and friends gather around the bride at a wedding. Most Ikarians belong to the Greek Orthodox Church, which has guided the pace of life on the island at least since the 17th century, when Joseph Georgirenes, the archbishop of Samos and Ikaria, wrote that "the most commendable thing of this Island is their Air and Water, both so healthful, that the People are very long liv'd."

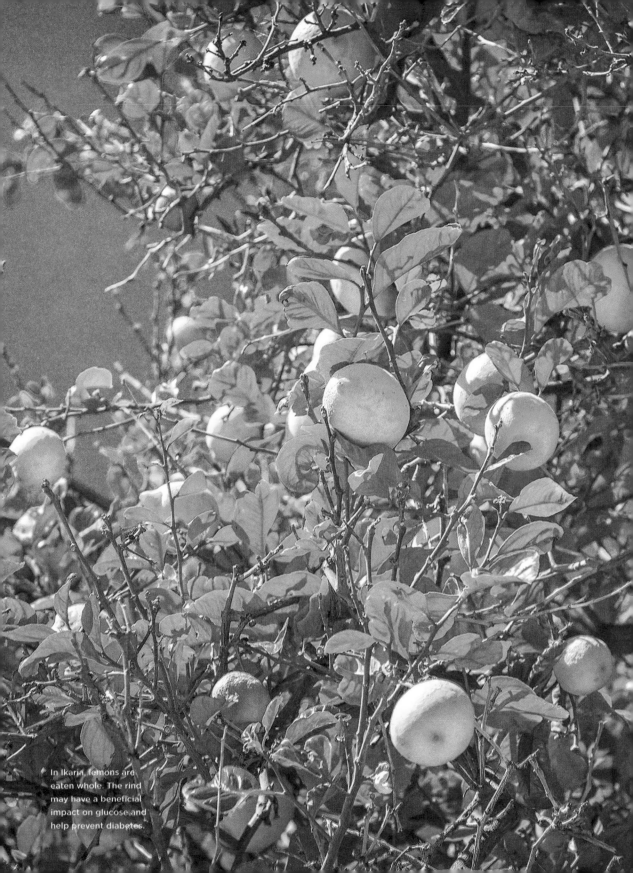

In Ikaria, lemons are eaten whole. The rind may have a beneficial impact on glucose and help prevent diabetes.

# Top Longevity Foods From Ikaria

Older Ikarians eat the purest form of the Mediterranean diet—heavier in beans and greens and lighter in fish and meat than other versions. Vegetables and greens, along with beans and fruit, account for 64 percent of their daily food intake, excluding dairy products and beverages like herbal tea. More than half the fat energy they consume comes from olive oil, which research associates with positive health factors. To enjoy the greatest benefit from olive oil, choose extra-virgin varieties. Keep a bottle on your table to drizzle over steamed or boiled vegetables.

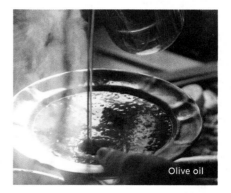

Olive oil

**BEANS** | Chickpeas, black-eyed peas, and other beans are eaten like a snack or added to soups or stews. Although chickpeas are high in fat, nearly all of it is unsaturated.

**FENNEL** | This herb, from bulb to seeds, is packed with nutrients, including calcium, iron, manganese, and potassium. Ikarians use it in cooking as well as in herbal teas.

**WILD GREENS** | Purslane, dandelion, arugula, and other wild greens are a great source of minerals as well as carotenoids, the colorful pigments the body converts to vitamin A.

**LEMONS** | Ikarians eat them whole, skin and all. The peel may have a beneficial impact on blood glucose, helping to control or prevent disease.

**OLIVE OIL** | Ikarians consume at least four tablespoons of olive oil a day, which may help protect them from heart disease. One study suggests it's also why Ikarians have a 50 percent lower mortality rate than Americans.

**OREGANO** | One of the many herbs used in Ikarian cooking, oregano is rich in antioxidants and compounds proved to help fight bacteria.

**POTATOES** | Ikarians eat them daily, unlike others who follow a Mediterranean diet. Studies suggest that potatoes can reduce blood pressure, fight diabetes, and prevent inflammation.

**HONEY** | Besides stirring it into coffee, older Ikarians also take a spoonful of honey in the morning and before dinner. It's also used to treat everything from colds to wounds.

**SAGE** | This herb may be one of the reasons that Ikarians have lower rates of Alzheimer's disease and dementia. It also has properties that help strengthen bones.

**ROSEMARY** | Used in herbal teas, rosemary has been shown to improve digestion and enhance memory.

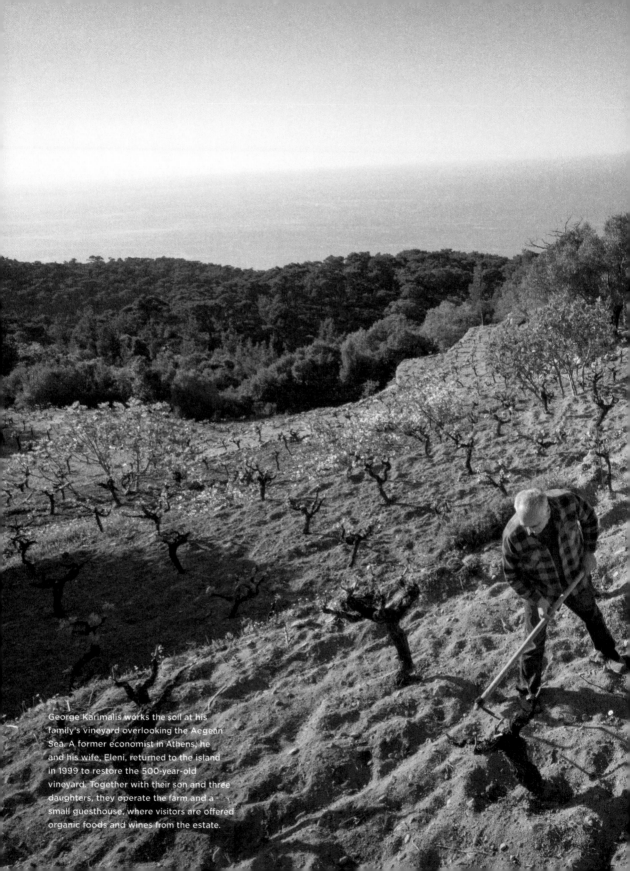

George Karimalis works the soil at his family's vineyard overlooking the Aegean Sea. A former economist in Athens, he and his wife, Eleni, returned to the island in 1999 to restore the 500-year-old vineyard. Together with their son and three daughters, they operate the farm and a small guesthouse, where visitors are offered organic foods and wines from the estate.

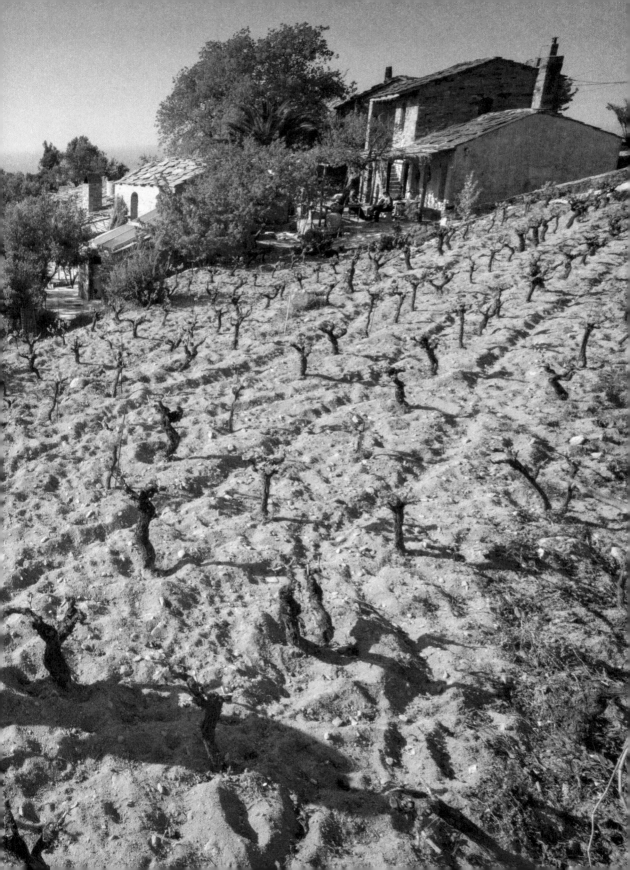

# LESSONS FROM IKARIA'S BLUE ZONE

■ **Mimic mountain living**

The longest-lived Ikarians tend to be poor. Residing on the island's steep terrain, they exercise daily by gardening, walking to their neighbor's house, or doing their own yard work. The lesson for you: Engineer more movement into your life.

■ **Eat a blue zones diet**

Ikarians eat a variation of the Mediterranean diet, with lots of fruits and vegetables, whole grains, beans, and olive oil—but with more potatoes, greens, and beans. Try sautéing—not frying—with olive oil, which contains cholesterol-lowering monounsaturated fats.

■ **Stock up on herbs**

People in Ikaria enjoy drinking herbal teas with family and friends, and scientists have found that those teas pack an antioxidant punch. Wild rosemary, sage, and oregano teas also act as a diuretic, which can keep blood pressure in check by ridding the body of excess sodium and water.

■ **Nap**

Take a cue from Ikarians and enjoy a midafternoon break. People who nap regularly have up to a 35 percent lower chance of dying from heart disease. It may be because napping lowers stress hormones or rests the heart.

■ **Fast occasionally**

Ikarians have traditionally been devout Greek Orthodox Christians. Their religious calendar calls for fasting almost half the year. Caloric restriction—a type of fasting that cuts about 30 percent of the calories out of a normal diet—is the only scientifically proven way to slow the aging process in mammals.

■ **Make friends and family a priority**

Ikarians foster social connections, which have been shown to benefit overall health and longevity. So get out there and make some plans.

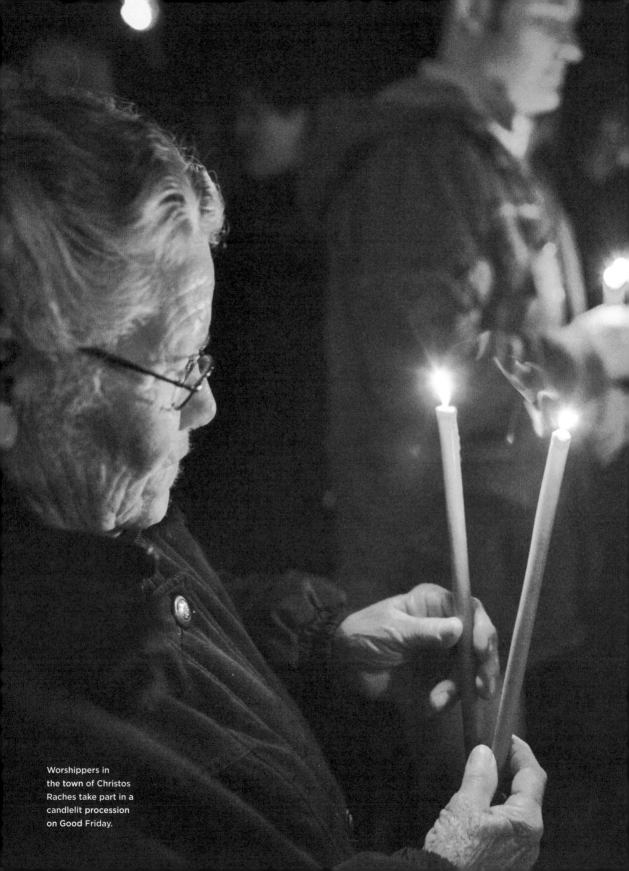

Worshippers in
the town of Christos
Raches take part in a
candlelit procession
on Good Friday.

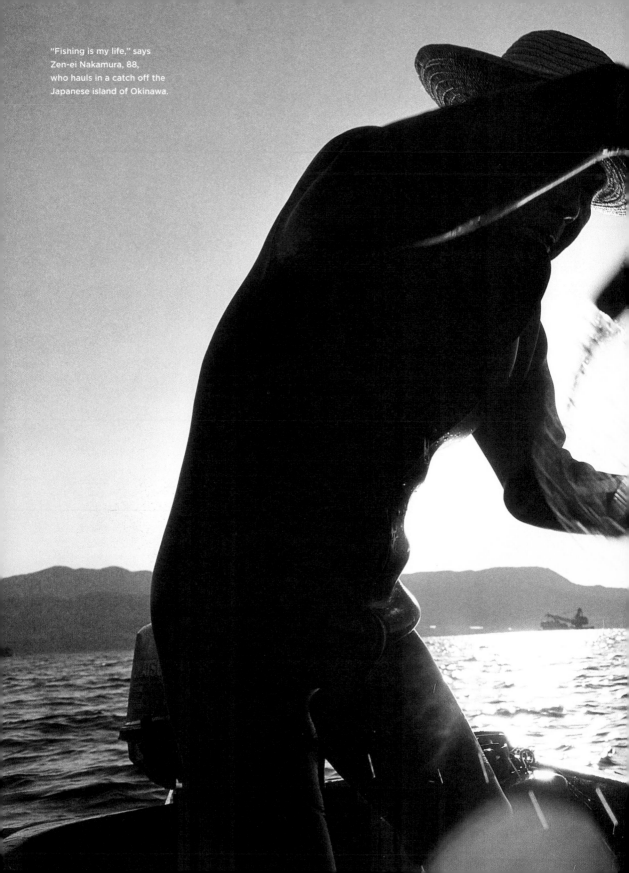

"Fishing is my life," says Zen-ei Nakamura, 88, who hauls in a catch off the Japanese island of Okinawa.

CHAPTER 5

# Okinawa

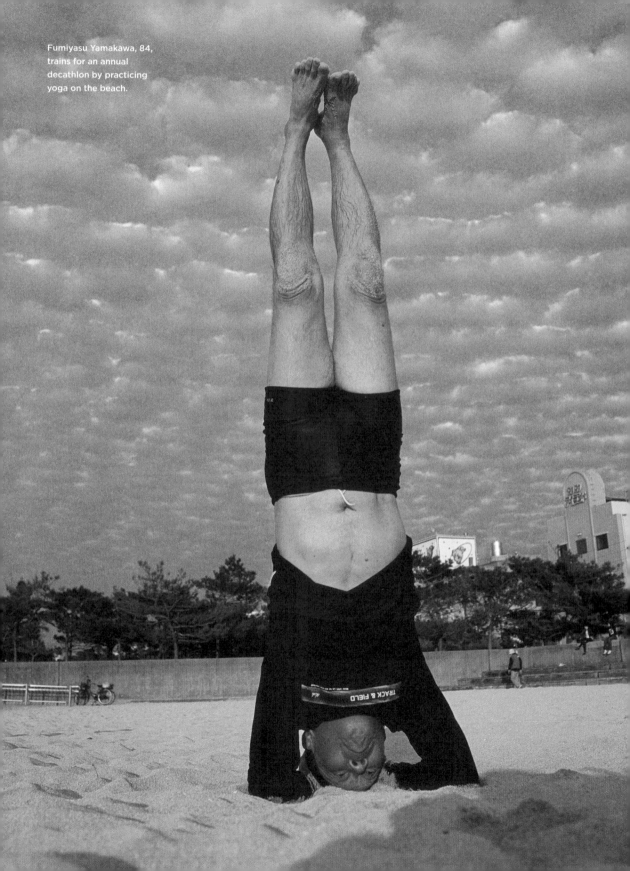

Fumiyasu Yamakawa, 84, trains for an annual decathlon by practicing yoga on the beach.

# A Fading Blue Zone

For almost a thousand years, the people of Japan's Ryukyu Islands have been known for their long lives. Chinese explorers who visited the archipelago centuries ago called it the "land of immortals," and until recently it has earned that reputation.

In fact, for decades the women on Okinawa, the largest island in the subtropical chain, have enjoyed the status of being the longest-lived women on the planet, with a life expectancy of 87.4 years—seven years more than American women. Okinawan men haven't lagged far behind, with a life expectancy of about 80.3 years, four more than American men.

As a group, Okinawans are three times more likely to reach the age of 100 than Americans—and to have far less disease in their later years. Okinawan women get breast cancer at about half the rate as American women, and both sexes have a fraction of the rates of heart disease and dementia from Alzheimer's as people in the United States.

And yet, for a while now the longevity phenomenon on Okinawa has been slipping away as younger generations abandon the lifestyle of their elders. In Japan's 2020 census, Okinawan women for the first time lost their top spot for health and longevity

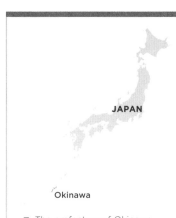

JAPAN

Okinawa

- The prefecture of Okinawa comprises 48 inhabited islands. About 95 percent of the population of 1.4 million lives on the main island of Okinawa.

- For decades, Okinawan women have been the longest lived in the world, with a life expectancy of 87.4 years—seven years more than American women.

- Okinawa is home to 55,000 U.S. military personnel and their family members.

among the nation's 47 prefectures, falling to seventh place. Okinawan men came in 36th.

What's going on?

The answer isn't hard to find. As you drive from the airport through Naha, the capital city, you muscle through snarled traffic and a concrete corridor of bunker-like buildings. This is partly a reflection of the city's typhoon-proof building strategy, but it's also a sign that Okinawan culture has been displaced by modern influences. It's difficult to find a traditional Okinawan restaurant in the city anymore. Instead, McDonald's, A&W Root Beer, TGI Fridays, Burger King, KFC, and Red Lobster dominate the eating environment.

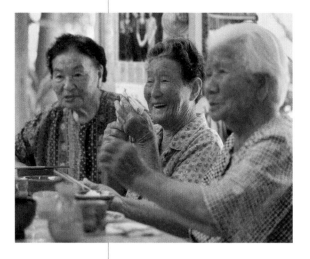

Laughter with good friends keeps minds sharp, prevents loneliness, and gives meaning to life for aging Okinawans.

That's what happens, I guess, when the inhabitants of a long, skinny island—15 miles across at its widest point—live among nearly 30,000 U.S. military personnel and their almost 25,000 family members for nearly eight decades. The islanders who emerged hungry and poor from famine and world war were suddenly surrounded by rich, processed foods. They developed a taste for Spam, the canned meat introduced by American GIs that the World Health Organization has put in the same category as smoking when it comes to promoting cancers. White rice replaced the more nutritious sweet potato that sustained the islanders for centuries.

Their new diet turned out to be toxic. Younger Okinawans now die from heart disease at a rate higher than most other Japanese do. The incidence of low birth weights on the island is 20 percent greater than in the rest of the country. And Okinawan men under 55 have the distinction of being the most obese in Japan.

The truth is, it's probably too late for this blue zone. When Okinawa's oldest generation is gone, the phenomenon of long life here will likely vanish with it. Which makes it even more urgent that we capture their recipe for successful aging while we can.

I've been visiting Okinawa since the spring of 1999. Back then, I was conducting one of my educational projects called "Quests." Along with a team of experts, I set out across the island to investigate the mystery of its long-lived residents guided by an online audience of roughly a quarter million schoolkids. The idea was that the students would vote each morning on whom we should interview that day and what questions we should focus on. And each night we'd sent back short videos and other reports of what we'd discovered. Remember, this was the early days of the internet. Facebook and Twitter didn't exist yet. During previous Quests, we'd ridden bikes across the jungles of Mexico, Belize, and Guatemala in search of an answer to why the ancient Maya civilization had disappeared. We'd dived into the waters off the Galápagos Islands to learn about environmental threats. We'd pedaled across China to find the real Silk Road.

This time, directed by our online audience, we set out to unravel the mystery of why Okinawans—at the time—enjoyed the world's longest disability-free life expectancy. We sat down with 13 centenarians on Okinawa and listened to their stories. They told us about their love of gardening, their reverence for their ancestors, and their diet rich in vegetables. We met with a ton of experts, as well, to gather more information, and by the end of our 10-day project we'd identified 18 "ingredients" in Okinawa's recipe for long life that students could put to use in their own lives.

Nearly 1,000 miles south of Tokyo, Okinawa Island is part of a subtropical archipelago.

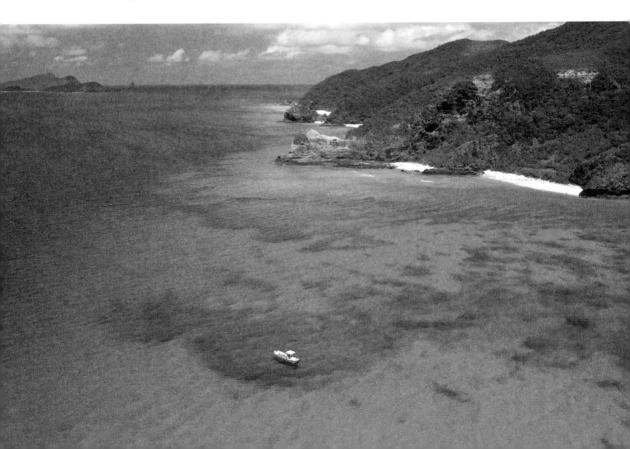

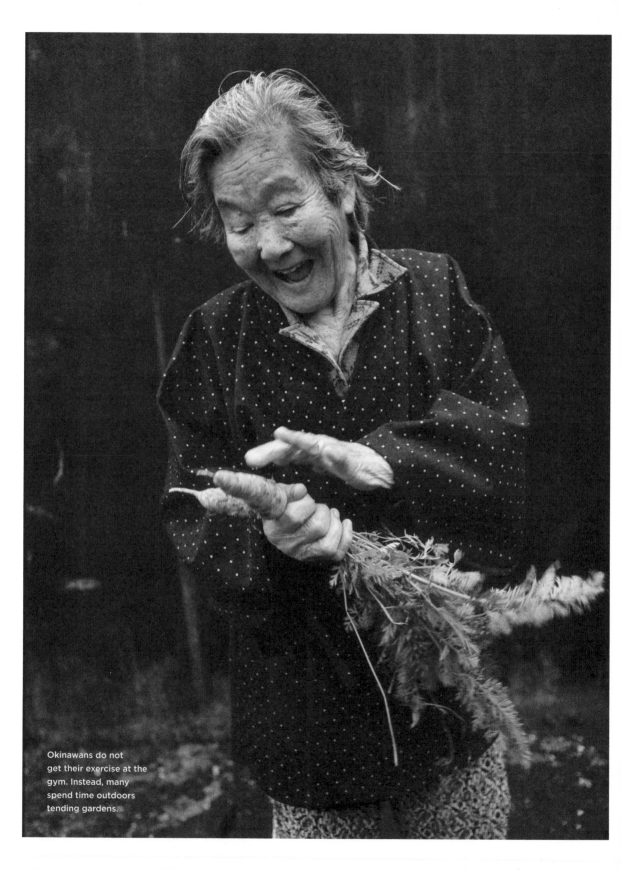

Okinawans do not get their exercise at the gym. Instead, many spend time outdoors tending gardens.

Since then, I've made regular visits to Okinawa, as curiosity about the world's blue zones has only increased, and I've often been accompanied by photographer David McLain. When David and I returned to the island in 2017 to research *The Blue Zones Kitchen* cookbook, my 85-year-old dad, Roger, came along for the ride. He grew up on a farm in rural Minnesota and recognized traditional Okinawans' penchant for hard work, gardening, pickling food, and living low off the hog, as it were. I figured his meat-and-potatoes upbringing would help us choose recipes for the book. So when he gave fermented tofu and blanched bitter melon (goya) the thumbs-down, we nixed them from the lineup.

In the village of Kunigami, at the northern end of the island, we met Miyo Oshiro, who took the three of us into her garden to show us what she was growing. Oshiro was well into her 90s, and yet she was amazingly agile, bending over to hoe and weed the soil. Even my dad was impressed. Afterward, she invited us back to her house, where she cooked us a meal of noodles with miso, garlic, and onions

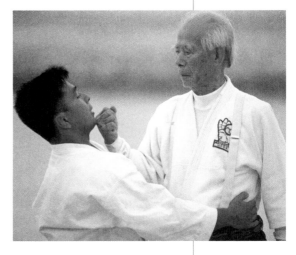

Passions such as karate give purpose to the lives of aging Okinawans.

from her garden, and my father, the quintessential Middle American, gave the dish a thumbs-up.

Like many of the blue zones women I've met over the years, Oshiro radiated a positive attitude and sense of purpose. More than that, she possessed an undeniable charisma—as have so many of the centenarians I've met here over the years. The first time I interviewed Kamada Nakazato, in 2005, the 102-year-old was wrapped in a kimono, her cottony, white hair brushed straight back, revealing high cheekbones and deep brown eyes. The moment we entered her house on the Motobu Peninsula, her eyes widened, and she gleefully raised her hands and began singing, swaying back and forth. Her children, both in their 70s, took the cue and clapped in unison with her. I felt an instant affection for her.

I noticed there was little furniture in Kamada's house except for a bed, which I learned was typical of Okinawan homes. Other than rollaway futons, cushions, and a low table for eating, they're completely uncluttered. This absence of furniture hazards accounts for fewer injuries and deaths among the

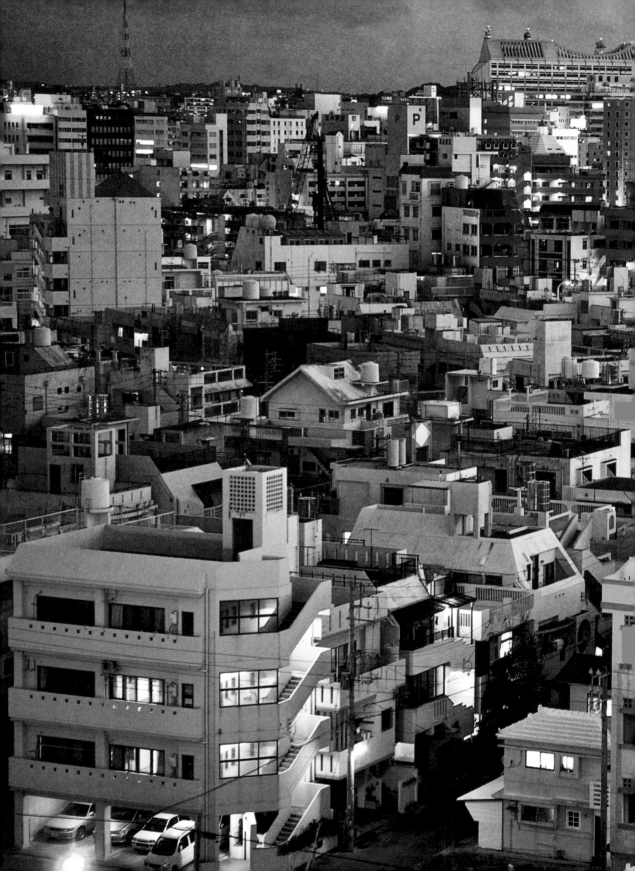

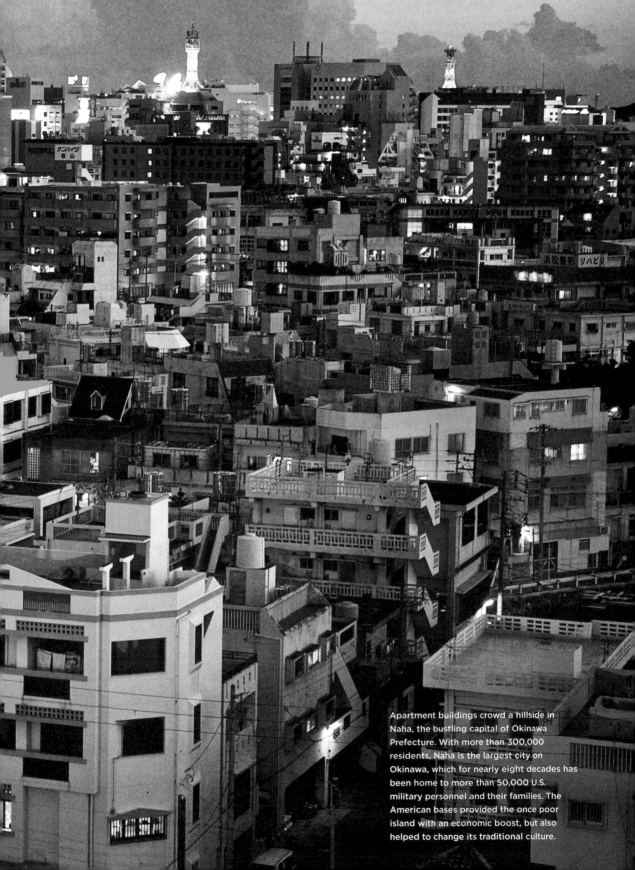

Apartment buildings crowd a hillside in Naha, the bustling capital of Okinawa Prefecture. With more than 300,000 residents, Naha is the largest city on Okinawa, which for nearly eight decades has been home to more than 50,000 U.S. military personnel and their families. The American bases provided the once poor island with an economic boost, but also helped to change its traditional culture.

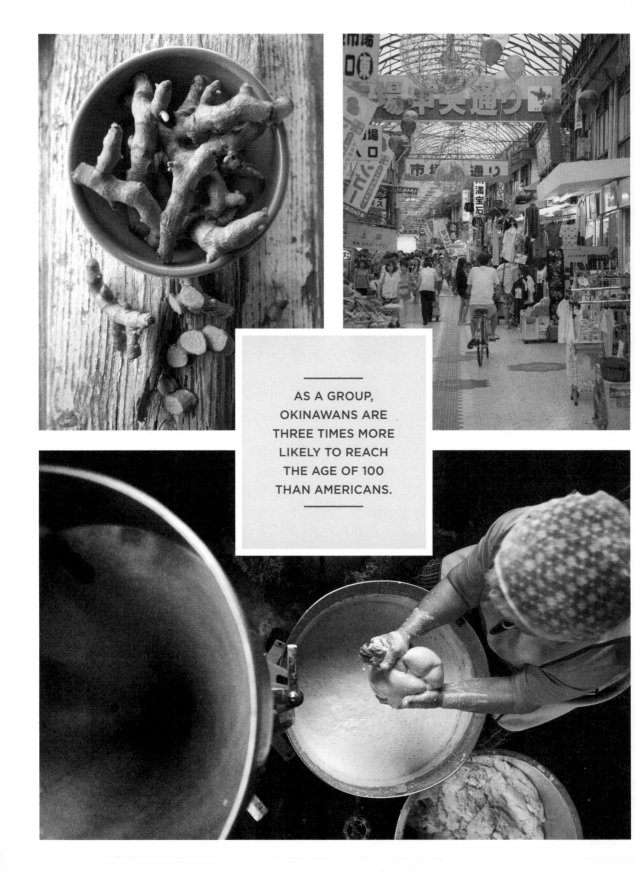

AS A GROUP,
OKINAWANS ARE
THREE TIMES MORE
LIKELY TO REACH
THE AGE OF 100
THAN AMERICANS.

elderly on the island, which is also the result of their high intake of sun-induced vitamin D, relatively low intake of medications, good balance, and high lower body strength. In contrast, falls are the leading cause of death among older Americans.

As the village *noro,* or priestess, Kamada told me she felt a deep responsibility for her community. "I go to the sacred grove to pray for the health of the village and thank the gods for making it safe," she said. The grove was a clearing in a nearby forest with a gazebo-like structure. There she communed with the gods and ancestors to help her carry out her duties as a spiritual adviser to the villagers. This was her *ikigai,* her reason for being.

When I asked Kamada for the secret to living beyond 100, she told me something I've remembered ever since. "I used to be very beautiful," she said. "I had hair that came down to my waist. It took me a long time to realize that beauty is within. It comes from not worrying so much about your own problems. Sometimes you can best take care of yourself by taking care of others."

"Anything else?" I asked.

"Eat your vegetables, have a positive outlook, be kind to people, and smile."

The blue zones recipe for living in a single short sentence.

Ushi Okushima was another of the first centenarians I got to know on Okinawa. When I met her in 2000, she lived in the tiny fishing village of Ogimi, and I can still hear her unmistakable laugh in my mind today. It began in the 104-year-old's belly, rumbled up to her shoulders, and then erupted with a hee-haw that filled the room with joy.

Ushi told me that she normally ate a diet of mostly vegetables, with a cup of mugwort sake before bed. Like most Okinawans her age, she'd grown up during a period of hardship, when many children went to bed hungry. There were even periods of famine when people starved to death. The one food they could count on was the *beni imo,* or Okinawan sweet potato, a purple variety related to the orange sweet potato that Americans know. Sometimes they ate imo for breakfast, lunch, and dinner. Fortunately for the islanders, it also happened to be one of the healthiest foods on the planet, with vitamin C, fiber, carotenoids, flavonoids, and slow-burning carbohydrates.

Opposite: (clockwise from top left): Turmeric— ginger's golden cousin—is a powerful antioxidant that Okinawans use in teas and soups. In a battle of modern culture and ancient traditions, Okinawa is both the home of crowded shopping arcades and a 73-year-old woman making tofu the traditional way.

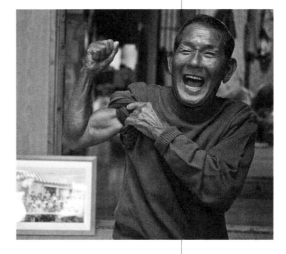

Above: Hard work and healthy foods have paid off for a fit 89-year-old fisherman.

In fact, as Bradley and Craig Willcox have documented in their decades of research, sweet potatoes provided more than 60 percent of the calories consumed by Okinawans before 1940. Bradley, a physician and resident scholar at the University of the Ryukyus, and Craig, a professor of public health and gerontology at Okinawa International University, wrote *The Okinawa Diet Plan*

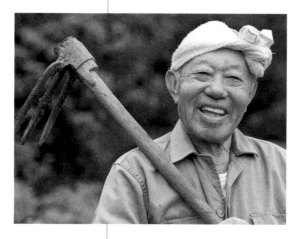

with Makoto Suzuki, who helped open Okinawa's first medical school in 1975. It was Suzuki who announced at an international conference in 1995 that he'd identified 40 centenarians on Okinawa, an extraordinarily high number for such a small place.

As the Willcoxes determined in subsequent studies, Okinawans traditionally consumed vegetables, small amounts of grain, soy in the form of tofu, the occasional egg, and fish when they could get it.

Hoei Tobaru, 90, works in his garden on Taketomi Island at the far southern end of the Ryukyu Islands.

The main dish in their traditional diet was *champuru,* or stir-fried vegetables, which might include goya, daikon radish, Chinese okra, pumpkin, burdock root, or green papaya. Rich in nutrients, but skimpy on calories, this diet was perfect for stimulating caloric restriction, a digestive survival mode that has verified longevity benefits. In a 2007 study the Willcoxes and their colleagues pointed out that Okinawans in their seventies consumed 10 to 15 percent fewer calories than normal from their youth to middle age. This was a result of their active lifestyle as farmers and their diet of nutrient-rich but energy-poor foods. The Willcoxes also speculated that specific foods in their diet, including

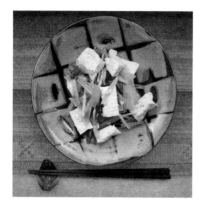

## OKINAWAN TOFU

Okinawans consume twice as much tofu as other Japanese, typically eating it twice a day. The traditional Okinawan version of this Japanese staple, called *shima* tofu, is firmer than the fluffier, unpressed type, called *yushi* tofu, that tends to be more popular in the rest of the country. That makes shima tofu ideal for most stir-fry recipes. Tofu is normally made from soybeans that are ground, boiled, strained, and pressed into shape. Low in fat and high in protein and calcium, tofu has been shown to reduce the risk of heart disease among vegetarians. Handmade tofu can be found in most towns on the island, where shops and supermarkets may even offer it still warm.

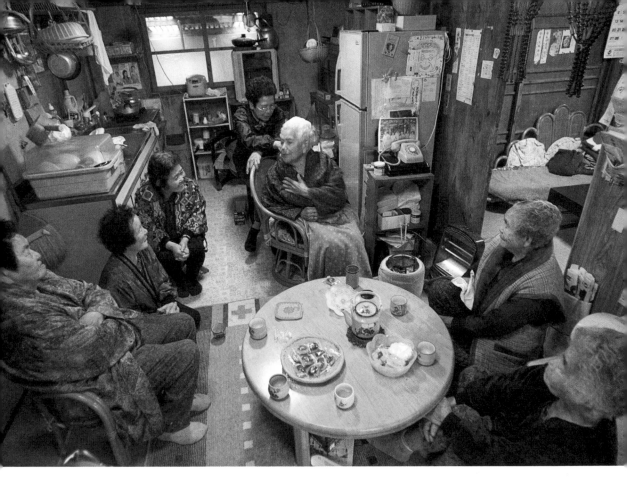

turmeric, sweet potatoes, and seaweed, also mimicked reduced calories in a way that delayed the aging process.

Something else that delayed aging among Okinawans was their tradition of helping one another through hard times. On the island of Uruma, just off Okinawa's main island, I dropped in on Mitsu Iha, Mitsuko Matayoshi, and Tomi Ito, who had belonged to the same *moai,* or committed social circle, for more than 40 years. During that time, they'd met with one another and other members of the group twice a month to pool small amounts of money and then give it to whoever was neediest at the time or just redistribute it. At one time, there had been 60 women in their moai, they told us, but now they were down to only 30.

The three women sat around a low table on a tatami mat, with a TV behind them and a group of ancestors staring down from a gallery of framed photographs on the wall. Some of the forebears had a 19th-century look, with their kimonos and army uniforms, while others gave off more of a 1970s vibe, with horn-rimmed glasses and Buddy Holly haircuts. When I remarked on the

Family and friends surround Kamada Nakazato, 102. Her advice for a long life: "Eat your vegetables, have a positive outlook, be kind to people, and smile."

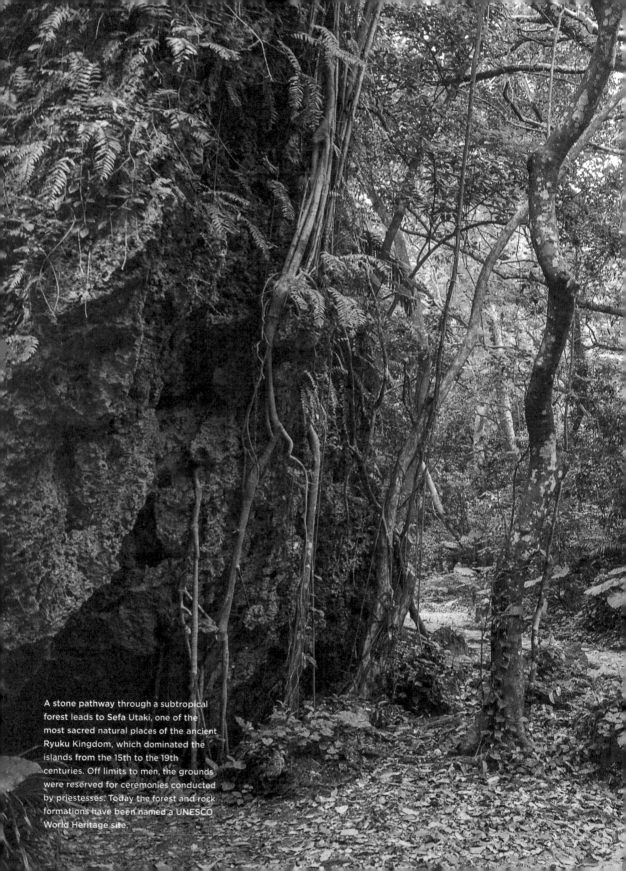

A stone pathway through a subtropical forest leads to Sefa Utaki, one of the most sacred natural places of the ancient Ryuku Kingdom, which dominated the islands from the 15th to the 19th centuries. Off limits to men, the grounds were reserved for ceremonies conducted by priestesses. Today the forest and rock formations have been named a UNESCO World Heritage site.

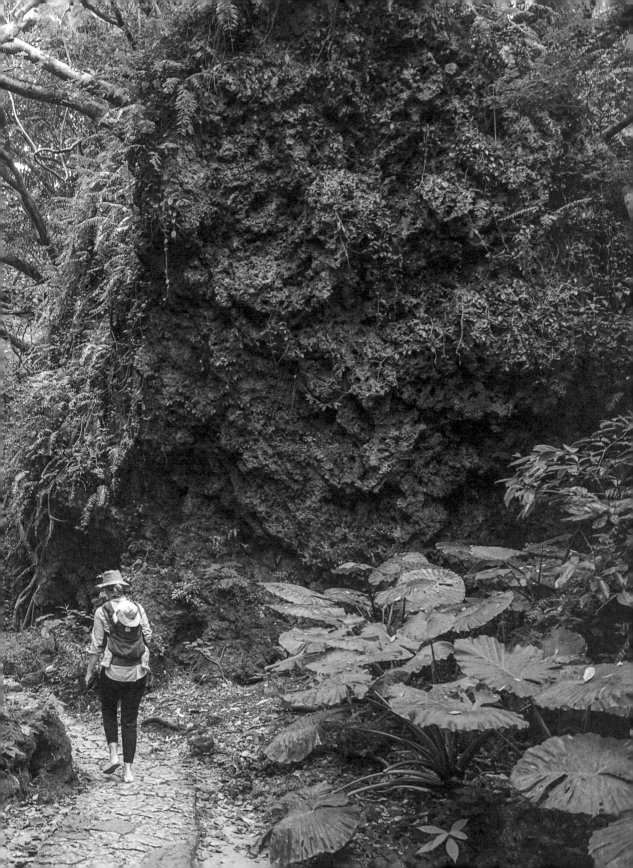

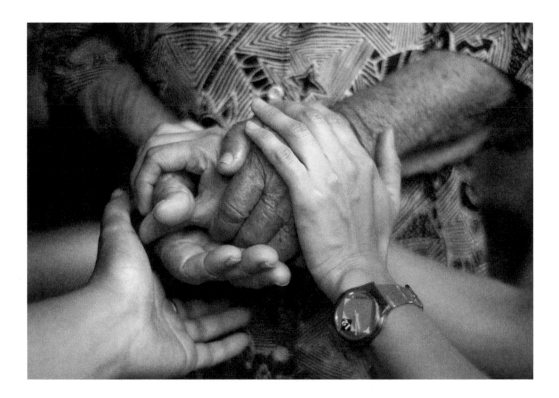

A centenarian holds the hands of her adult grandchildren, whose love and support have added years to her life.

location of the portraits, the women laughed and said the photos were up there so the ancestors could watch the TV.

I knew that Okinawan moais had originally served as financial backups. Back in the day, peasants didn't have access to bank loans. Belonging to a moai might enable a farmer to buy seed or a mother to pay medical bills for her sick child. And yet, as I watched the women banter with one another, it was clear that their moai had served an important social purpose as well, keeping them from being lonely and encouraging them to stay active well into old age.

Did they agree that their moai had contributed to their longevity, I asked?

The women stared at me, perplexed. No, we just hang out all the time, they said.

It would be difficult to overestimate the hardship women of their generation had been through. During World War II, when most Okinawan men were conscripted into the Japanese army and U.S. warships bombarded the island, many women fled into the mountains with their children, where they survived on berries or whatever else they could scavenge. An estimated 80,000 Okinawan women, children, and older men hid in caves from the fighting that began on April 1, 1945, when U.S. forces invaded. Within 82 days, a third of

# Tofu Steak With Mushrooms

TOTAL COOK TIME: 20 MINUTES • SERVES 2

This recipe is adapted from the Okinawa Program (a plan authored by the scientists of the Okinawan Centenarian Study), but we asked Sensei Yukie Miyaguni, head of a cooking school in Okinawa, to spice it up. This is a perfect main dish that will delight vegetarian friends and even satisfy meat eaters. Soybean-based foods, including miso and tofu, are key staples in the traditional Okinawan diet, which is high in nutrients and antioxidants but low in calories and fat.

½ pound firm tofu, sliced into four rectangular pieces

1 tablespoon all-purpose flour

1 tablespoon vegetable or soybean oil

1 tablespoon sesame oil

1½ cups shiitake mushrooms, sliced

1 tablespoon mirin

1 teaspoon grated ginger

1 tablespoon red miso paste

½ teaspoon red pepper flakes

½ cup chopped leeks or green onion

4 cherry tomatoes, halved for garnish

In a medium bowl, coat the tofu with the flour.

In a sauté pan over medium-high heat, brown the tofu in the vegetable or soybean oil for 3 to 4 minutes per side.

In a separate pan, heat the sesame oil over medium heat. Add the mushrooms, mirin, ginger, miso, and pepper flakes and sauté for 3 to 4 minutes, or until the mushrooms are cooked.

When done, turn off the heat and add the leeks or green onion to the pan, mixing to combine.

Place two pieces of tofu per plate and cover with the seasoned mushrooms.

Garnish with cherry tomato halves.

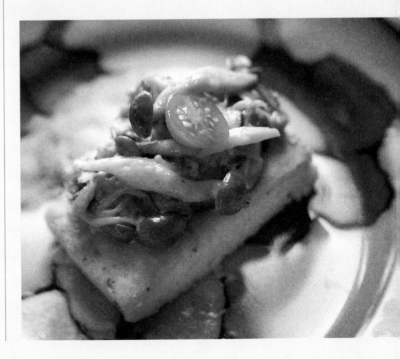

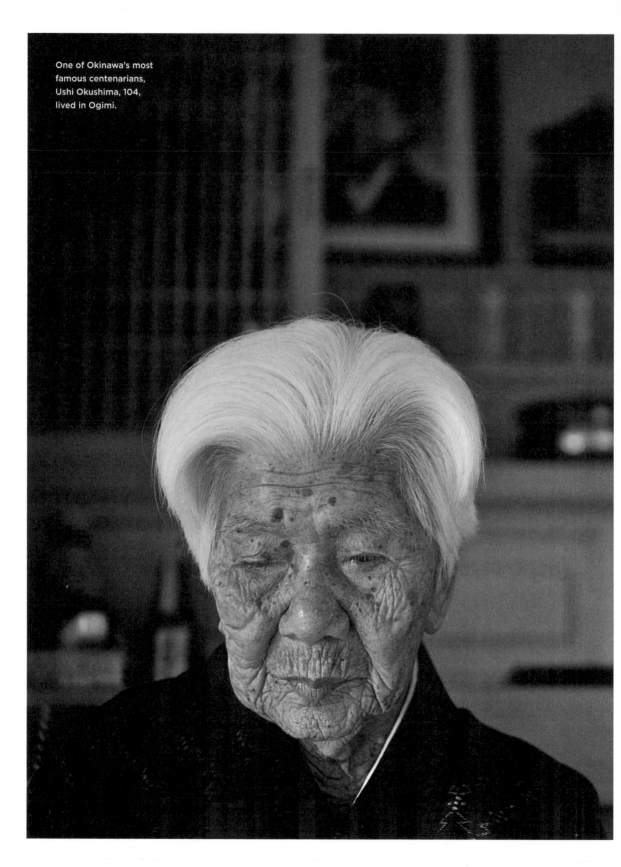

One of Okinawa's most famous centenarians, Ushi Okushima, 104, lived in Ogimi.

the island's population—between 100,000 and 150,000 civilians—were dead, along with 12,520 Americans, and 110,000 Japanese soldiers and Okinawan draftees. It was the largest battle in the war in the Pacific.

The conflict was hard on everyone, said Miyo Oshiro, when I caught up with her again this past spring. Standing about four and a half feet tall, she walked with two canes now. Since the last time we'd spoken, her daughter had come home to care for her.

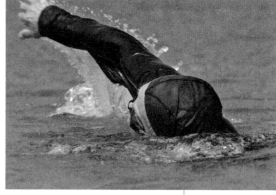

Oshiro recently had been honored at a *kajimaya* celebration. When Okinawans turn 97, they're often celebrated with a special party. The word *kajimaya* translates to "windmill," a reference to the cyclical nature of life. Those who reach 97 are thought to have completed many cycles of experience, gathering wisdom along the way, returning finally to the innocence of childhood. There's even a special red kimono for the ceremony. But Oshiro told her family she'd had a dream in which she wore a wedding dress for her ceremony. They said, "Fine, for your kajimaya, you can wear a white wedding dress, if you want to."

Besides doing yoga on the beach every morning, 84-year-old Fumiyasu Yamakawa also swims in the ocean off Naha, Okinawa.

She cried again as she shared this with us. Our visit had prompted her to recall memories, both good and bad, from her long life, and I marveled at her generation's ability to put behind them a painful past and live in the moment.

After a long pause, she smiled. "This is the most memorable day of my life."

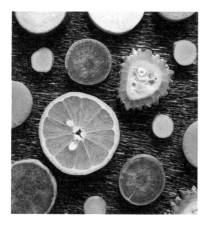

## OKINAWAN SUPERFOODS

Some of the brightest stars in the Okinawan constellation of longevity foods come from the family garden, including the purple sweet potato known as *beni imo*, which contains high quantities of antioxidants; and turmeric, a golden cousin of ginger that Okinawans consume as both a spice and a tea, which provides anti-inflammatory agents. Green disks of bitter melon, known as goya, come from a long knobby gourd often called for in recipes of Okinawan *champuru*, a stir-fry dish. An island staple, bitter melon is also believed to act as an antidiabetic food that regulates blood sugar. Compared with American foods, Okinawa's plant-based diet is rich in nutrients but light on calories.

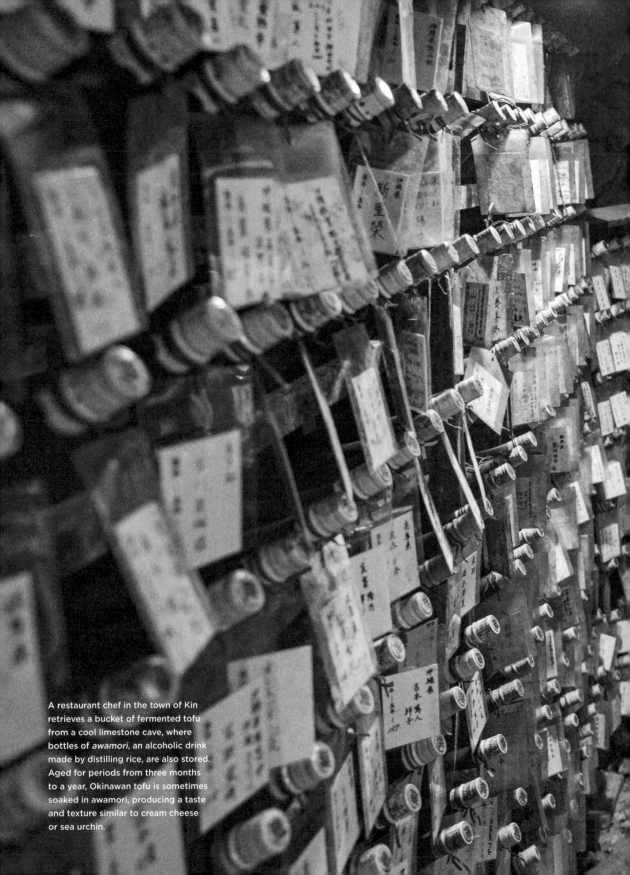

A restaurant chef in the town of Kin retrieves a bucket of fermented tofu from a cool limestone cave, where bottles of *awamori*, an alcoholic drink made by distilling rice, are also stored. Aged for periods from three months to a year, Okinawan tofu is sometimes soaked in awamori, producing a taste and texture similar to cream cheese or sea urchin.

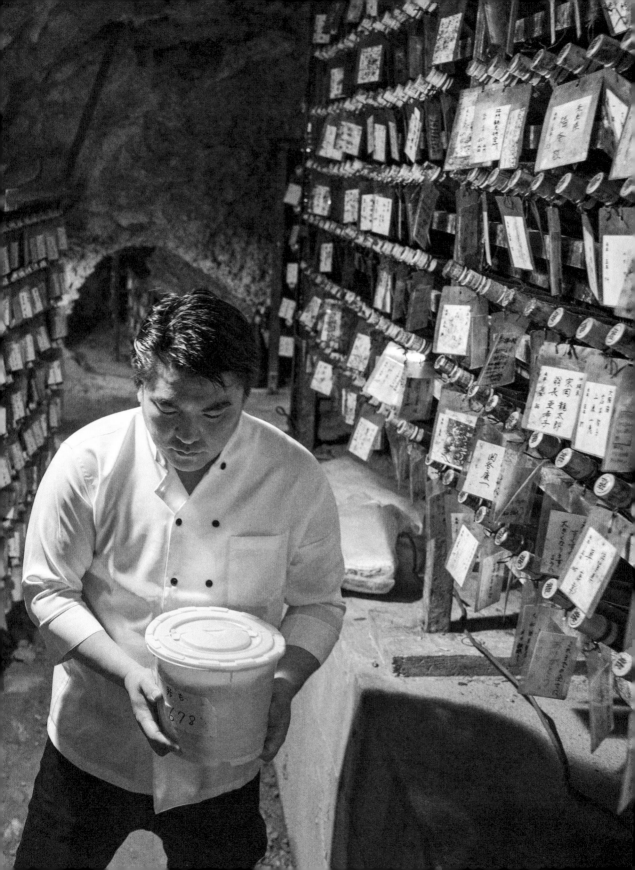

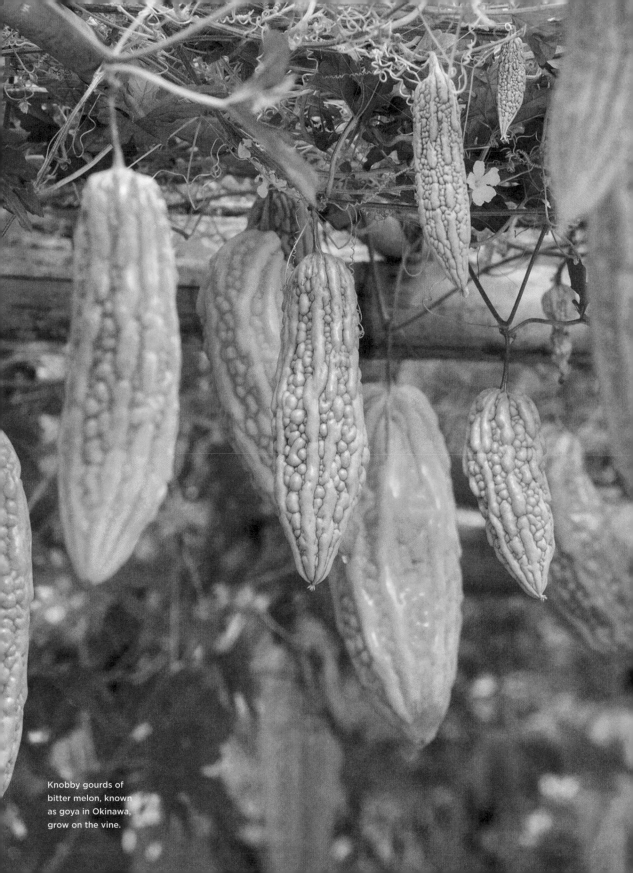

Knobby gourds of bitter melon, known as goya in Okinawa, grow on the vine.

# Top Longevity Foods From Okinawa

During the first third of their lives, most Okinawan centenarians obtained the majority of their calories from the purple or yellow sweet potato known as the imo. Related to the orange variety Americans know, the imo is one of the healthiest foods on the planet—high in vitamin C, fiber, carotenoids, flavonoids, and slow-burning carbohydrates. They also tended to eat more meat, primarily pork, than other Japanese, but less fish, less salt, and less added sugar. In recent decades, a Western diet of fast and processed foods has replaced traditional foods, causing Okinawa to slide significantly from its top spot.

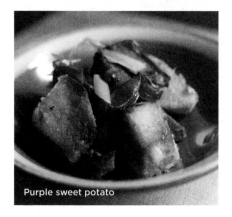

Purple sweet potato

IMO | A supercharged sweet potato, imo doesn't cause blood sugar to spike as much as a regular white potato does.

DASHI BROTH | This soup is rich in amino acids, which are fundamental to keeping your body healthy.

GREEN ONIONS | An excellent source of vitamins K and C, green onions can be used from top to bottom.

MISO | Rich in various vitamins, miso is fermented and provides loads of beneficial gut bacteria.

SESAME OIL | High in zinc and copper, sesame oil is known to boost heart health and improve circulation.

BITTER MELON | Known as goya, bitter melon is an effective antidiabetic food and helps regulate blood sugar. It is also the base of many *champuru*, or stir-fry, dishes.

SEAWEED AND KELP | Rich in carotenoids, folate, magnesium, iron, calcium, and iodine, seaweed and kelp provide a filling, low-calorie nutrient boost to the diet.

MUSHROOMS | Shiitake and other mushrooms contain more than 100 compounds with immune-protecting properties.

TOFU | Okinawans eat tofu like the French eat bread. Studies show that people who eat soy products in place of meat have lower cholesterol and a lower risk of heart disease.

TURMERIC | Ginger's golden cousin, turmeric is a powerful anticancer, antioxidant, and anti-inflammatory agent.

# LESSONS FROM OKINAWA'S BLUE ZONE

■ **Find your** *ikigai*

Older Okinawans can readily articulate the reason they get up in the morning. Their purpose-imbued lives give them clear roles of responsibility and feelings of being needed well into their 100s.

■ **Rely on a plant-based diet**

Older Okinawans have eaten a plant-based diet most of their lives. Their meals of stir-fried vegetables, sweet potatoes, and tofu are high in nutrients and low in calories. Goya, or bitter melon, with its antioxidants and compounds that lower blood sugar, is of particular interest.

■ **Eat more soy**

The Okinawan diet is rich in foods made with soy, such as tofu and miso soup. Flavonoids in tofu may help protect the heart and guard against breast cancer. Fermented soy contributes to a healthy intestinal ecology and offers even better nutritional benefits.

■ **Garden**

Almost all Okinawan centenarians grow or once grew a garden. It's a source of daily physical activity that exercises the body with a wide range of motion and reduces stress.

■ **Build your** *moai*

The Okinawan tradition of forming a moai provides secure social networks. These safety nets lend financial and emotional support in times of need and give all their members the stress-shedding security of knowing that there is always someone there for them. To build your own, see page 231.

■ **Enjoy the sunshine**

Vitamin D helps produce stronger bones and healthier bodies and reduce the chance of depression. Spending time outside each day allows older Okinawans to have optimal vitamin D levels year-round.

■ **Activate your home environment**

Older Okinawans are active walkers and gardeners. In Okinawan households residents take meals and sit on tatami mats on the floor. The fact that old people get up and down off the floor dozens of times daily builds body strength and balance.

■ **Plant kitchen herbs**

Mugwort, ginger, and turmeric are all staples of an Okinawan garden, and all have proven medicinal qualities. Okinawans grow herbs right in their kitchens. By consuming these every day, Okinawans may be protecting themselves against illness.

■ **Be interested and interesting**

Older Okinawans possess a generosity of spirit and likability that draws people to them. Quick to offer a cup of tea and a snack to visitors, they ask questions and seem happy to share their life stories.

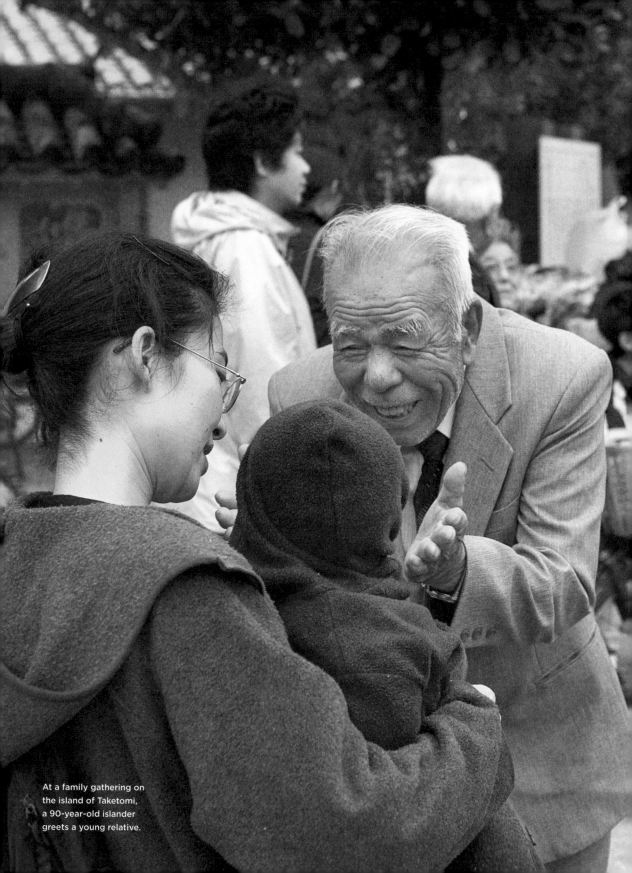

At a family gathering on the island of Taketomi, a 90-year-old islander greets a young relative.

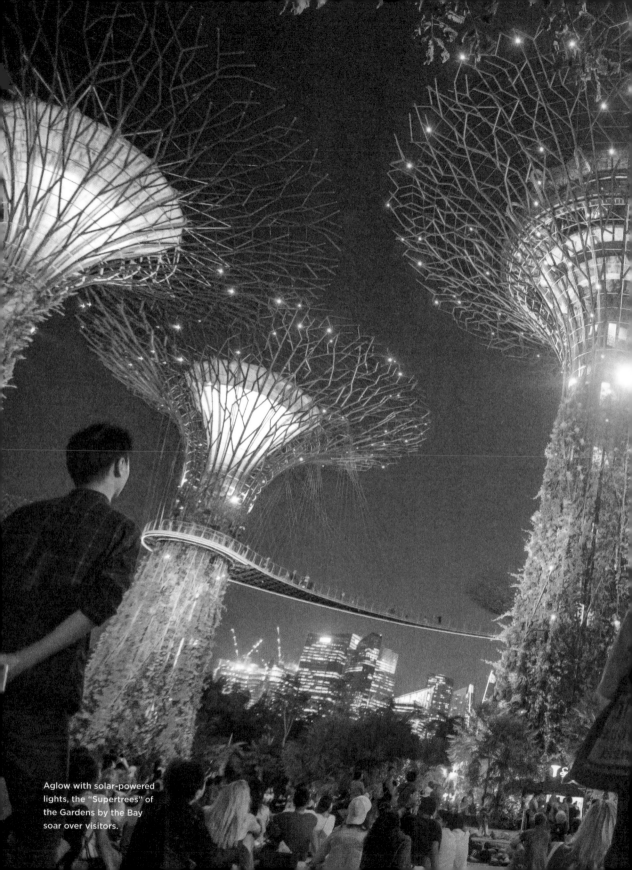

Aglow with solar-powered lights, the "Supertrees" of the Gardens by the Bay soar over visitors.

# CHAPTER 6

# Singapore

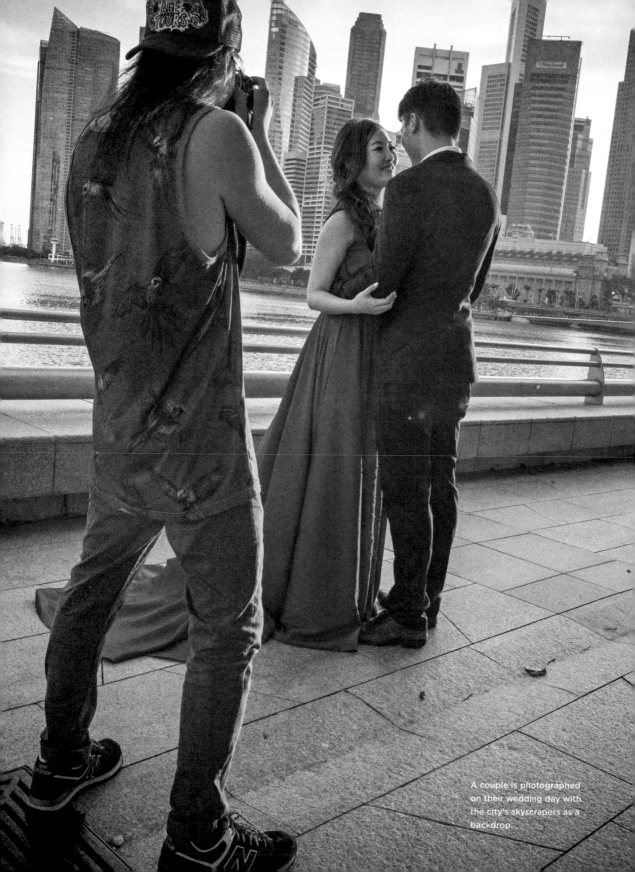

A couple is photographed on their wedding day with the city's skyscrapers as a backdrop.

# Blue Zone 2.0

Douglas Foo arrived in style. Gliding to a stop in front of my hotel in his black BMW i8, he popped open the gullwing door of his sleek hybrid sports car and emerged in his customary blue tailored suit, a radiant smile on his face.

"Ready to roll?" he asked.

With boundless enthusiasm and irrepressible energy, Foo epitomized the Singaporean ideal of success. In 1997, at age 28, he founded Sakae Sushi, a fast-food chain that now has more than 200 restaurants globally. In his spare time, he volunteered with dozens of charities and business groups and even served as a nominated member of Singapore's parliament. And yet, when I asked him a few years ago if he was proud of his accomplishments, he told me that he still wasn't satisfied.

"Singapore has given me so much, and I don't do enough to give back," he said.

Foo's tiny, ambition-driven nation, less than six decades old itself, can also seem like a bundle of paradoxes at times. Since its founding in 1965, Singapore has transformed itself from a large fishing village into a complex urban society with thousands of high-rises and more than 150 shopping malls serving 5.8 million residents. Its highly educated, multi-ethnic citizenry is a blend of Chinese, Malay, and Indian populations.

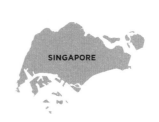

**SINGAPORE**

- Only a fourth the size of Rhode Island, Singapore is home to nearly 6 million people.

- About 74 percent of Singaporeans are ethnically Chinese; 13 percent are Malay; and 9 percent are Indian.

- The Port of Singapore is one of the busiest in the world.

- Government policies shape the lives of most citizens.

While famous for its draconian laws governing behavior as trivial as spitting or chewing gum, Singapore ranks among the world's healthiest, happiest, and longest-lived places on the planet. And it wasn't always that way.

In 1960, the average newborn in Singapore could expect to live only 65 years. Now, one lifetime later, life expectancy has grown by almost 20 years. Of all the nations in the world, it ranked number one in 2019 for life expectancy at birth, at 84.9 years, six more years than in the United States. What's more important, Singaporeans rank number one in healthy life expectancy and have the world's lowest rate of cardiovascular mortality and best health-care system. The number of centenarians on the island more than doubled during the past decade, from 700 to 1,500, as did the number of men and women in their eighties and nineties. Clearly, Singapore has been doing something right for its aging population—and doing it in its own way.

Unlike the other blue zones, Singapore was no isolated region where a traditional culture evolved a lifestyle of longevity over a period of centuries. Instead, it was a busy crossroads of commerce and cultures whose leaders from the start set out to *create* an environment of health and well-being. In fact, you might even call it a blue zone 2.0—the next frontier of aging.

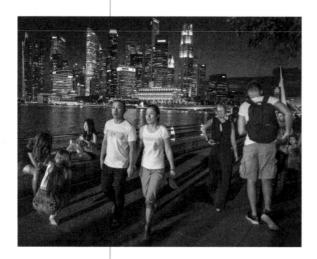

Even at night, families feel safe strolling along the Singapore River on pathways near Esplanade Park.

"Hop in, we're late," Foo said, after bidding me a good morning. He was taking me to Yishun, a town on the northern side of the island, to visit Khoo Teck Puat Hospital, where, of course, he served on the board of directors.

KTPH, as it's known, opened with great fanfare in 2010 as a facility that would "lower one's blood pressure" just by entering its forestlike grounds. Lauded for its innovative design, it immersed patients in a soothing natural environment with lush vegetation spilling over its balconies, a cascading waterfall, and expansive rooftop gardens, among other features.

To me, the place looked more like a Four Seasons hotel than like a hospital. In fact, as we strolled the breezy lower level, Foo told me the staff had consulted luxury hotels when they designed the rooms, as well as Singapore Airlines when they planned the food service.

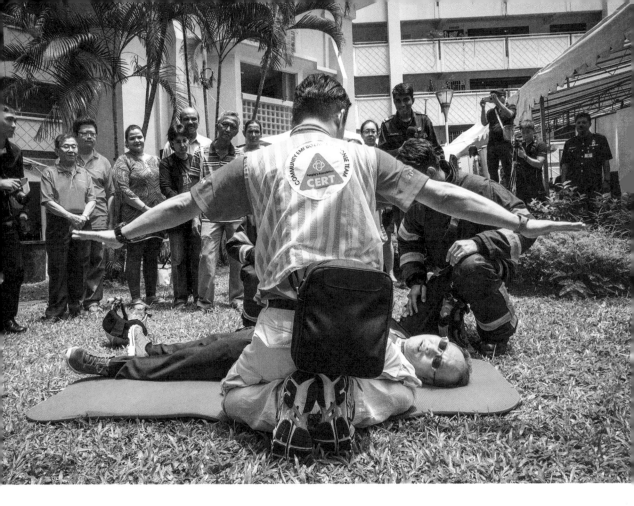

A member of the Community Emergency Response Team demonstrates first aid for neighbors.

And it wasn't just for the patients and staff, either. The hospital also aimed to draw in the surrounding community. The public was encouraged to enjoy the grounds, too, and to eat at the hospital's health-oriented restaurants and to take part in tai chi and Zumba classes. People from the neighborhood enjoyed their lunches in picnic areas, while patients in wheelchairs were pushed through an artificial tropical rainforest, instead of languishing in their hospital rooms. Up on the roof, local volunteers tended a 2.5-acre garden that produced organic vegetables, herbs, and fruit for both patients and the public.

Foo led me through the soaring main lobby to meet Dr. Wong Sweet Fun, a deputy chairman of the medical board who oversaw initiatives for the elderly. A thin woman with a welcoming smile, she spoke about the hospital's outreach with evangelical zeal.

The basic problem, she said, was that people in Singapore were living longer, but their final years weren't especially healthy ones. Women on the island tended to suffer through 13 years with a chronic illness such as heart

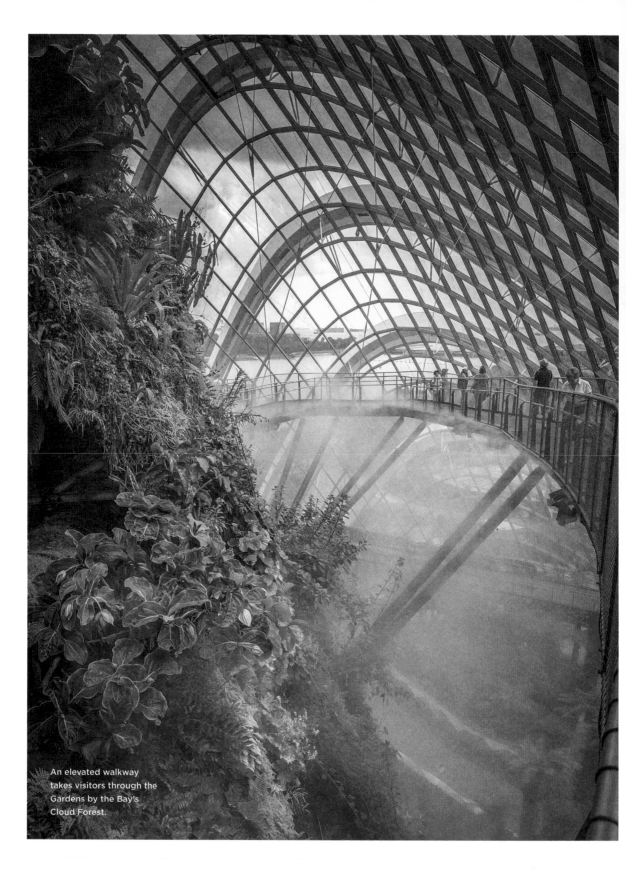

An elevated walkway takes visitors through the Gardens by the Bay's Cloud Forest.

disease, diabetes, or cancer, while for men it was 10 years. The main causes were poor diets, sedentary lifestyles, and stress. The hospital's goal was to turn these around with prevention, education, and lifestyle changes.

"If someone is living with a chronic disease, we don't make them come to us," she said. "We go to them."

The hospital dispatched nurses into the community to conduct free screenings and talk to residents. They connected people living by themselves with others in the community and held cooking classes for healthy recipes. One of Wong's favorite initiatives was the Share a Pot program, in which volunteers bought discounted vegetables at the market for soup. Other volunteers did the cooking. Seniors were invited to a community center or school for a free meal, a little exercise, and a checkup. In the process, they made some new friends.

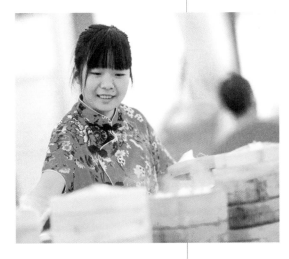

"We didn't focus on their frailty," she said. "We focused on what was strong in them. We emphasized dignity, not charity."

As I already knew, Singaporeans as a whole were fairly healthy. In Bloomberg's annual index of the world's healthiest nations, the island routinely ranked in the top 10. Compared with the United States, which came in 35th in the 2022 index, Singapore at number 8 spent only a fraction of its GDP on health care, even though it managed to provide health services to more than 92 percent of its population.

A girl samples food at a Lunar New Year party.

Still, when I spoke to officials at the Health Promotion Board, which is responsible for preventive health care on the island, they told me Singapore needed to do better.

"Like many other public health agencies, we focused on education at first," said Shyamala Thilagaratnam, the outreach director. "But that didn't work as well as wanted. So we decided to change the environment instead, to make the healthy choice easier."

Working with soda companies, they reduced the amount of sugar in sweetened beverages sold in Singapore. They enlisted restaurants to serve healthier foods and put "Healthy Choice" labels on products at the supermarket that contained less sugar, fat, or sodium. At the same time, they promoted

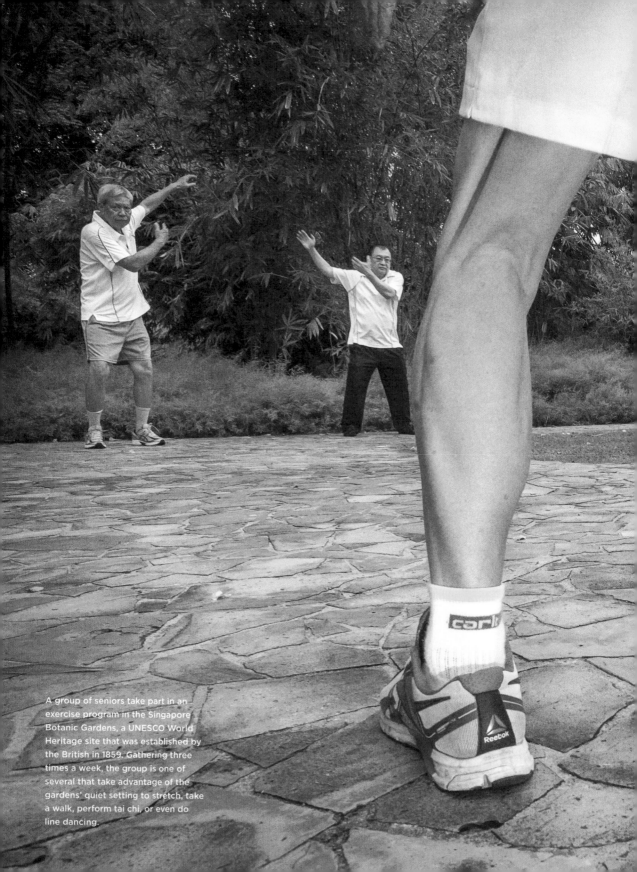

A group of seniors take part in an exercise program in the Singapore Botanic Gardens, a UNESCO World Heritage site that was established by the British in 1859. Gathering three times a week, the group is one of several that take advantage of the gardens' quiet setting to stretch, take a walk, perform tai chi, or even do line dancing.

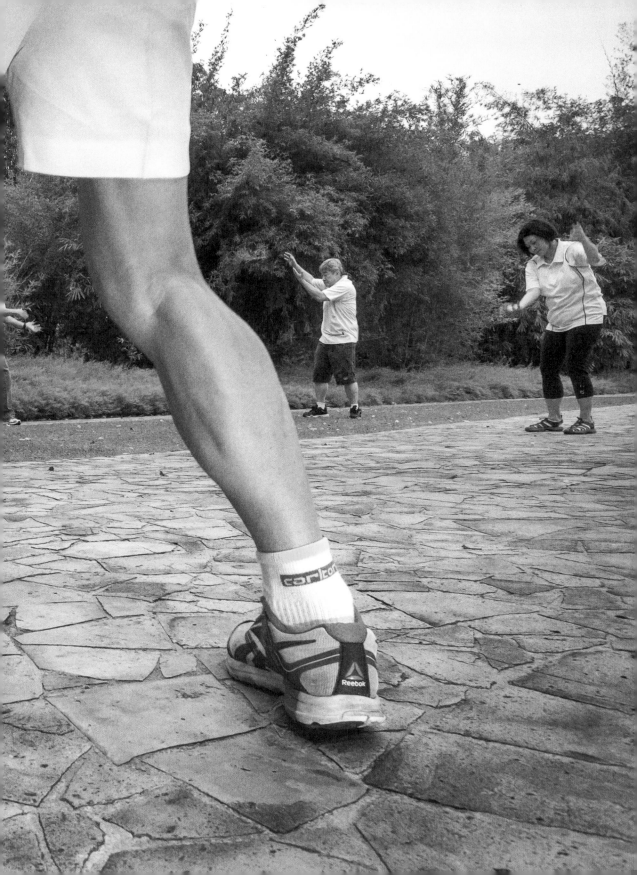

greater vegetable consumption and subsidized the supply of brown rice.

One of the most popular new ideas was the National Steps Challenge, which turned exercise into a game. Anyone who logged 10,000 steps a day on their mobile device qualified for Healthpoints that they could redeem for vouchers to spend at restaurants, movies, or public transportation, among other options. Now in its eighth year, the challenge has attracted more than 1.7 million people to take part.

Nobody had to bribe the "silver seniors" to work out. I met a trio of would-be musclemen, all in their seventies, in the playground of a public housing complex. It was a steamy morning, and the place was abuzz with activity. One of the guys had a perfectly round shaved heard, a workout outfit, and the hardened determination of someone tempered by military service. The second had a full head of silver hair and wore a light blue T-shirt and wire-framed glasses that telegraphed a certain pensiveness. The third had thinning black hair and bandy legs, and looked rather older than his friends.

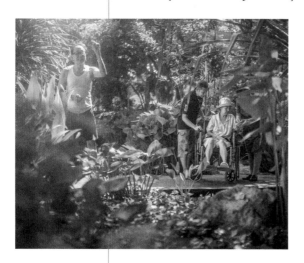

Surrounded by soothing tropical plants, patients and family members feed the fish in the green spaces of Khoo Teck Puat Hospital.

They came to the park every day, they told me. To prove it, the guy with the shaved head did the splits, while the others laughed. They could not only do more pull-ups than I could, they claimed, but they could also hold a plank for a minute.

The guy with the glasses said he'd come from China, where they didn't focus as much on physical fitness. When he moved to Singapore, he said, he started to work out more, because public housing complexes provided exercise areas that made it easier.

When I pushed them, they admitted that their desire to stay fit was only part of their reason for showing up every day. They also valued their friendship. When I asked if they owned cars, only the guy with black hair said he did, but he didn't use it much.

"How do you get around, then?" I asked.

"We take the bus or the subway," said the guy with glasses. "Or we walk."

After some gentle cross-examination, they calculated that they each walked between 8,000 and 14,000 steps a day—more than twice as many as the average American—which seemed to surprise them.

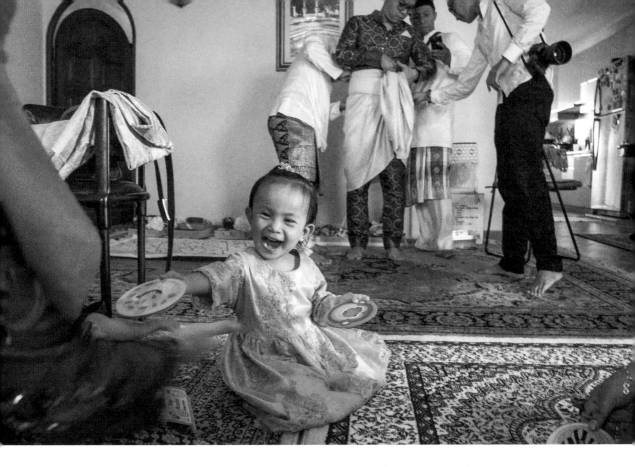

"So you probably get as much exercise from walking as you do from working out in the park," I suggested.

They gave me skeptical looks that suggested I'd missed the point. They didn't walk for exercise. They did it because everybody in Singapore did it. Walking was normal.

This was no accident. Like almost everything in Singapore, it was the result of a deliberate policy. To make the city more pedestrian-friendly, the government had invested in covered walkways—more than 125 miles of them since 2018—to provide relief from the blazing sun and tropical rains. They provided sidewalks where people felt safe and a fast, cheap, and efficient subway and light-rail system no more than a quarter mile from anyone's house. Leafy trees and garden-like foliage covered more than 45 percent of Singapore, and a world-class system of 350 parks circled the island, bringing a park within a 10-minute walk of 90 percent of the population. When someone in Singapore wanted to go to the store, go out to eat, or visit a friend, they usually did so on foot.

Of all the ways that Singapore has tried to shape the environment to promote healthy living, one of the most impressive I've come across was a senior housing project called Kampung Admiralty. Built in 2018, it's located on a former naval base—hence the "Admiralty" part of its name—and it was inspired by the concept of a *kampung*, or Malay village. The idea was to surround seniors with nature and other people.

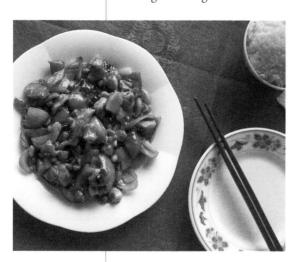

Like most buildings in Singapore, the 11-story complex was packed in among other high-rises. But when I stepped inside, I entered a breezy, open plaza on the ground floor that lifted my spirits. Along with a supermarket and retail shops, there's an area set aside for exhibitions or other community events, a stage for performances, and floor space for Zumba and tai chi classes. People of all ages and ethnicities circulated through the place as if in an indoor park.

An escalator took me to the second floor, where I found a hawker center, or food court, with vendors selling Malay *prata* (flatbread), Chinese stir-fries, and Indian curries. The center was open to the public, but on this day the tables were full of ethnically diverse older folks who'd probably come down from their apartments on the upper floors. They were playing dominoes or chatting over tea.

Waiting for me at a small table was the lead architect of the project, Pearl Chee. With a warm smile and shoulder-length black hair, the 40-something described the novel way she and her team had gone about creating a place where generations would meet.

"We took a club-sandwich approach," she said.

Because of the relatively small footprint they had to work with—only two and a half acres—they stacked everything vertically in three basic layers. The first included the plaza and food court I'd already seen. Above us on the third and fourth floors was the medical-center layer, with facilities for doctor's visits and minor surgery. The third layer was a community park, where generations could meet—or at least bump into each other. A preschool and elder care center sat side by side, with a playground tucked into a tropical garden nearby.

Flanking the park were castle-like towers containing 104 apartments for seniors with age-appropriate designs and emergency rip cords to signal for

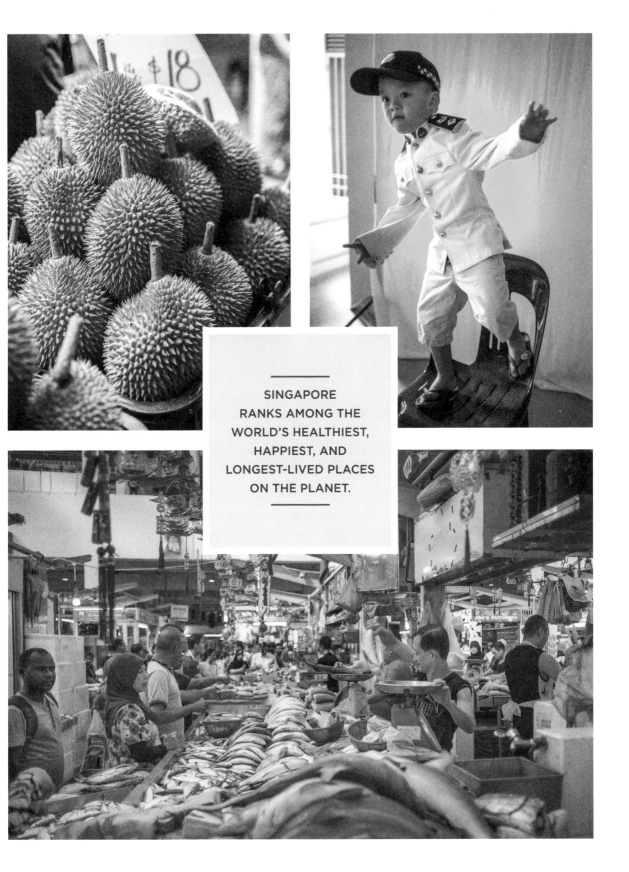

SINGAPORE
RANKS AMONG THE
WORLD'S HEALTHIEST,
HAPPIEST, AND
LONGEST-LIVED PLACES
ON THE PLANET.

# Vegetarian Singaporean Chili "Crab"

TOTAL COOK TIME: 20 MINUTES • SERVES 2

Singaporean chili crab, originated by chef Cher Yam Tian in the 1950s, is largely considered the national dish of the island nation. Found throughout Southeast Asia, the dish is typically made with hard-shell crabs (in Singapore, they use mud crabs), stir-fried in a sweet-and-spicy tomato sauce. This version has all the flavors of the rich, thick sauce but uses tofu as a plant-based alternative to crab.

1 tablespoon cornstarch

2 tablespoons extra-virgin olive oil

2 tablespoons grated ginger

4 garlic cloves, minced

4 bird's eye chilis, minced

1 green onion, finely chopped, plus more for garnish

½ cup tomato paste

¼ teaspoon white pepper

1 tablespoon sugar

1½ cups vegetable broth

2 cups cubed tofu, patted dry

½ cup chili garlic sauce

In a small bowl, whisk the cornstarch and 2 tablespoons of warm water and set aside.

Warm the olive oil in a large sauté pan over medium-high heat. Add the ginger, garlic, chilis, and green onion. Stir until fragrant, about 30 seconds, being careful not to burn.

Add the tomato paste, white pepper, and sugar to the pan. Stir until mixed thoroughly and a thick paste begins to form, about 2 to 3 minutes.

Pour the vegetable broth into the pan and bring to a simmer.

Add the tofu to the mixture and stir to coat. Simmer for 5 to 10 minutes, or until the tofu is warmed through.

Add the chili garlic sauce and simmer for 1 minute. Add the cornstarch slurry and mix well. Bring to a boil and allow the mixture to thicken, stirring frequently, about 3 to 4 minutes.

Ladle into bowls and serve warm, garnished with green onion.

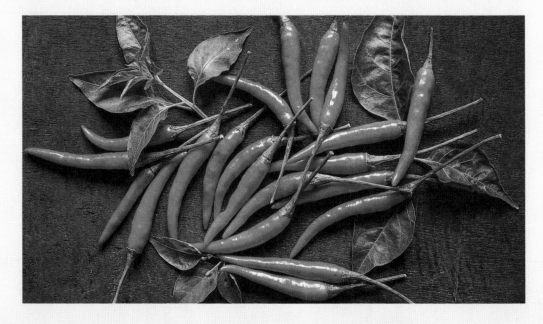

help from the medical facilities below. "Buddy benches" were strategically located to stimulate interaction among neighbors. Community gardens invited residents to get outside and connect with nature.

To pull off a project as ambitious as Kampung Admiralty, her team needed to satisfy a wide range of stakeholders, Chee said. I could only imagine the bureaucratic red tape. And yet, Singaporeans seemed to possess a special talent for collaboration. To me, what she and her group had accomplished was the best example I'd seen on the island so far of a manufactured blue zone environment where different generations could connect and live out their sense of purpose.

So, what was it about Singapore—and its people—that made such bold efforts possible? Could we learn from their methods to improve our own lives? For an answer I turned to one of the nation's best-qualified individuals. From 1996 to 2012, Chan Heng Chee was Singapore's ambassador to the United States. In that post, she acquired a unique insight into the similarities and differences between the two countries.

I met former ambassador Chan at her office at Singapore University, where she was a professor at the Lee Kuan Yew Centre for Innovative Cities. At

Volunteers conduct a cooking class for seniors living at a public housing facility to promote healthy active aging.

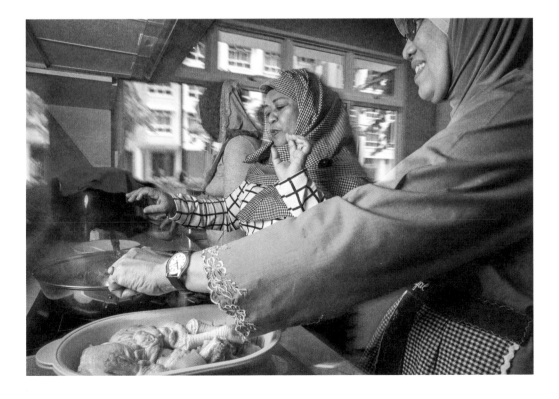

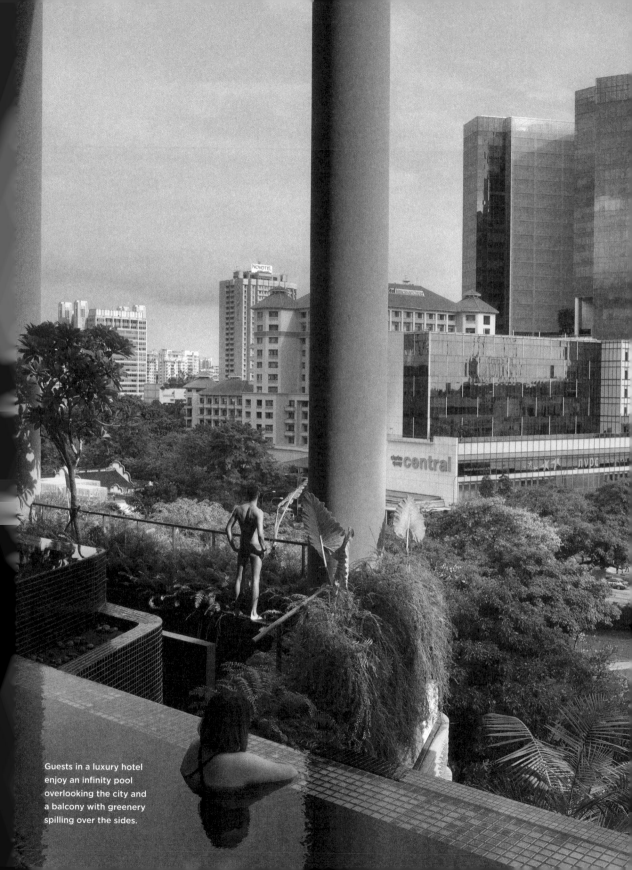

Guests in a luxury hotel enjoy an infinity pool overlooking the city and a balcony with greenery spilling over the sides.

age 80, she spoke with clarity and candor about her nation's strengths and challenges.

"We're a small nation. There's little room for mistakes," she said. "So we're forced to have strategic thinking."

That's why people in Singapore tended to talk policy all the time. There was a policy for everything, and the public generally went along with it. "Not because we are a compliant people," she said. "It's a bit of a show-me society. 'You tell me to do this— what's your proof?'" So politicians lay out the facts and trust the public to grasp them.

In the late 1990s, officials recognized that the nation's population was graying, she said. By 2030, a fourth of the people were expected to be over the age of 60. This being Singapore, they knew that would

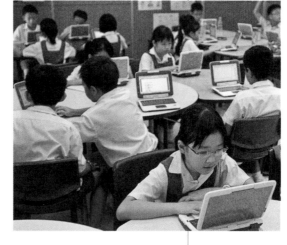

The education system is highly rated in Singapore, where primary school students work on their computers.

create a financial crisis. So beginning around 1999, there was this multi-ministerial focus on aging. All the ministries came together—finance, health, housing—and figured out a nationwide plan where everybody was on the same page. The result was a range of new programs and subsidies aimed at health-care insurance and support.

Which didn't mean there was no dissent in Singapore. In a complex multi-ethnic society, where so much emphasis was placed on getting ahead and making money, tensions and stress were unavoidable. Especially stress.

But when it came to following their leaders, Singaporeans were largely on

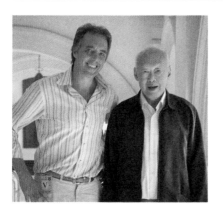

## LEE KUAN YEW

Considered by many the nation's founding father, Lee Kuan Yew was a young lawyer in 1965 when he led Singapore's movement to gain independence from Malaysia. Knowing the island had few natural resources, he promoted policies to turn Singapore into a trade and financial hub. At the same time, he strived to create a society that was efficient, orderly, well educated, and tolerant, famously endorsing strict punishment for crimes. His aim was to maintain harmony among the nation's Chinese, Malay, and Indian populations by offering them stability and a chance to achieve wealth. He died in 2015 at the age of 91.

board. In a recent poll, 70 percent said they trusted their government, compared with only 39 percent of Americans who responded to the same survey.

I heard clear echoes in Chan's words of an interview I conducted years ago with Lee Kuan Yew, the man widely regarded as Singapore's founding father. It was 2009, and I'd been invited to the retired leader's secluded five-acre compound. Expecting a stiff, formal interview with an intimidating disciplinarian, I was greeted instead with a warm smile from an 86-year-old in casual slacks, loafers, and a Mister Rogers sweater.

As a young politician in the late 1950s, Lee had pushed for Singapore's independence from British rule. Elected the country's first prime minister, he and his team led the country's rapid transformation into a financial powerhouse.

One of the world's largest aquariums, the S.E.A. Aquarium on Sentosa Island has more than 100,000 sea creatures on display.

I asked him what he was thinking back then. Did he have a plan from the start to lay the groundwork for a healthy, happy population?

"It was simpler than that," he replied. "I had to make it work, or we'd all die."

Their little island had no natural resources, so they needed to make themselves relevant to the rest of the world, he explained. "That relevance was

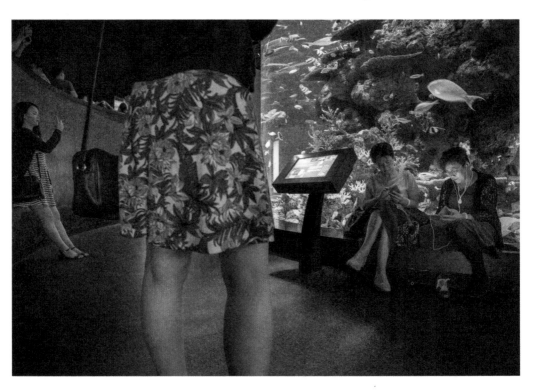

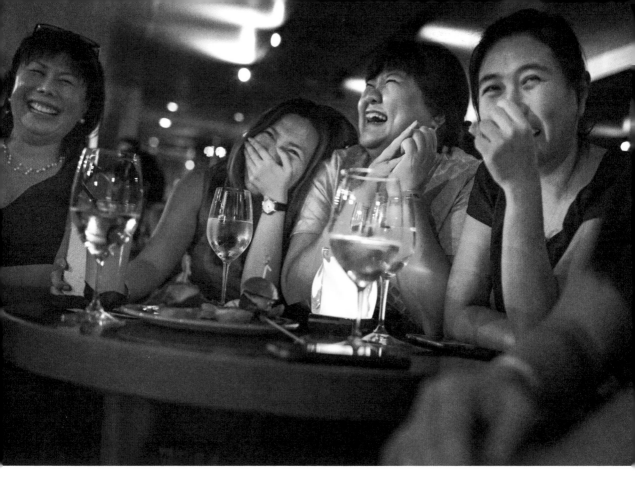

economics: our efficiency, our ability to provide a base for secure production, commerce, services, exploration of business opportunities in the region, logistics hubs, transportation of people and goods, in every possible way."

To help connect with the world of commerce, they decided to make English the official language in Singapore. This also helped avoid rivalry among the nation's Chinese, Malay, and Indian populations. He assured religious freedom for these same groups and made it possible for everyone to obtain an apartment in public housing, while mandating a proportional mix of ethnic groups in each high-rise.

At the same time, Lee's government set out to create a society that was efficient, orderly, well educated, and tolerant. They offered subsidies for education, housing, and health while insisting that citizens also earn their own way—even those at the bottom. Anybody who made an effort to work, no matter how lowly the job, was guaranteed a livable wage. "We call it workfare, not welfare," he said. "We say, we'll give you this, but you work. You earn your keep, and we will 'top up.'"

Workers from a paint company enjoy a laugh together during an employee appreciation event.

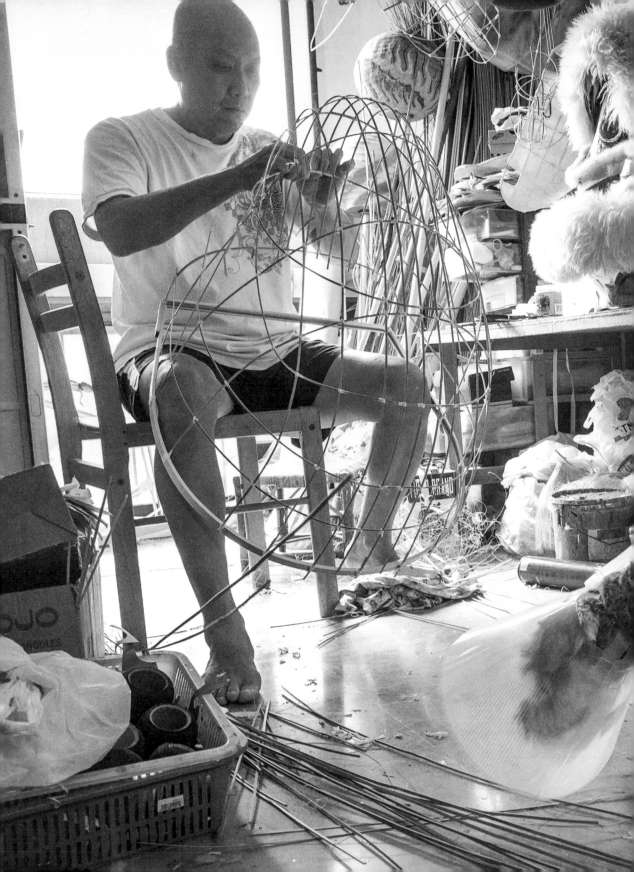

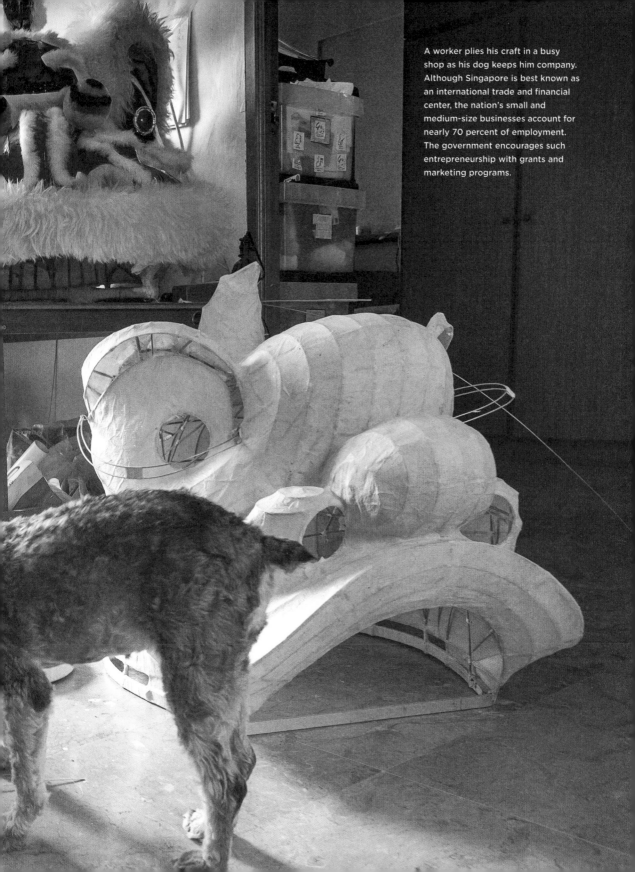

A worker plies his craft in a busy shop as his dog keeps him company. Although Singapore is best known as an international trade and financial center, the nation's small and medium-size businesses account for nearly 70 percent of employment. The government encourages such entrepreneurship with grants and marketing programs.

This deliberate leveling of society—economically, socially, and health-wise—was part of Lee's plan, in other words. "We went out of our way to make sure we didn't have an upper class," he said. "But you also won't see beggars in Singapore. You won't see ghettos."

To outsiders, the government's heavy hand seems nowhere more visible in the punishment of minor crimes such as littering or vandalism. Marijuana and vaping are also outright illegal. Indeed, all narcotics are illegal, with possession of 15 grams of opioids carrying the death penalty. This may sound draconian, but in 2021 only 17 people died of narcotics overdoses in Singapore. In the United States the number exceeded 100,000, a toll that doesn't account for the collateral damage of broken families, crime, and loss of productivity. So, which system is more compassionate?

Similarly, guns are strictly illegal in Singapore. No one except the police and military can own them. In 2021, 57,000 Americans died in gun violence. In Singapore the number was three. Guns and drugs are not just social issues, since they also materially impact life expectancy.

There was a light rain the morning I caught up with Crystal Thong at Clarke Quay on the Singapore River. She wore a hooded raincoat over her red-checked blouse, jeans, and galoshes. With her black hair and mom glasses, she looked 10 years younger than her 82 years.

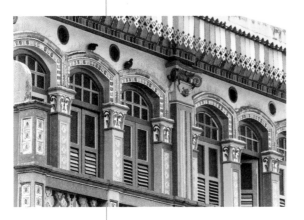
Vibrant colors enliven shops in the Little India neighborhood of downtown Singapore.

## LOVE TO SHOP

With more than 150 malls in their tiny city-state, Singaporeans have turned shopping into a national sport. From the busy markets of Chinatown (right) to the upscale boutiques of the Shoppes at Marina Bay Sands, conspicuous consumption is on full display. Encouraged by government policies, Singaporeans believe in working hard, saving money, investing wisely, and building wealth, creating one of the highest GDPs in the world, with one in 30 adults becoming a millionaire. At the other end of the economic ladder, Singapore's "workfare" program ensures that basic necessities such as housing and health care are covered for everyone.

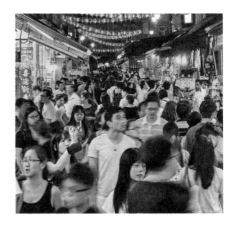

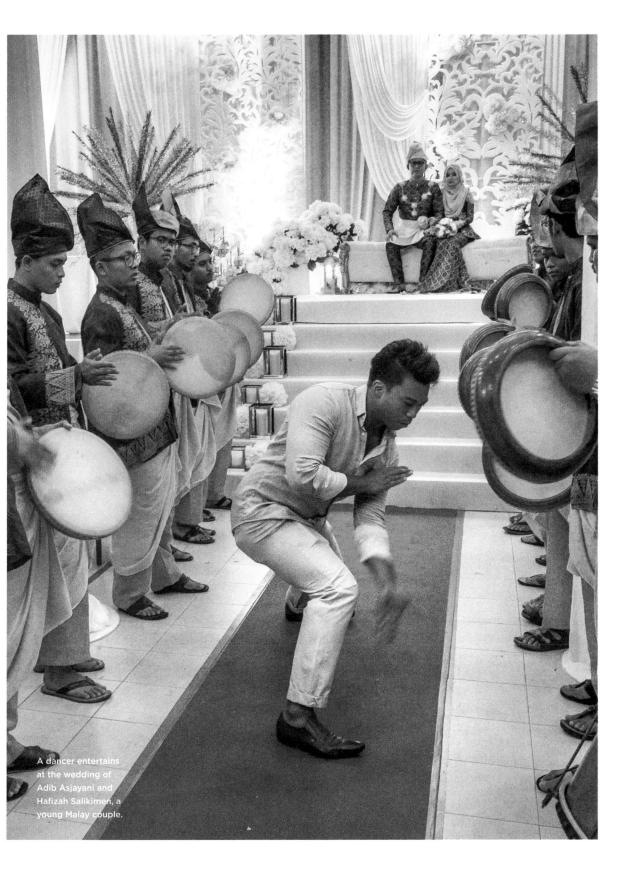

A dancer entertains at the wedding of Adib Asjayani and Hafizah Salikimen, a young Malay couple.

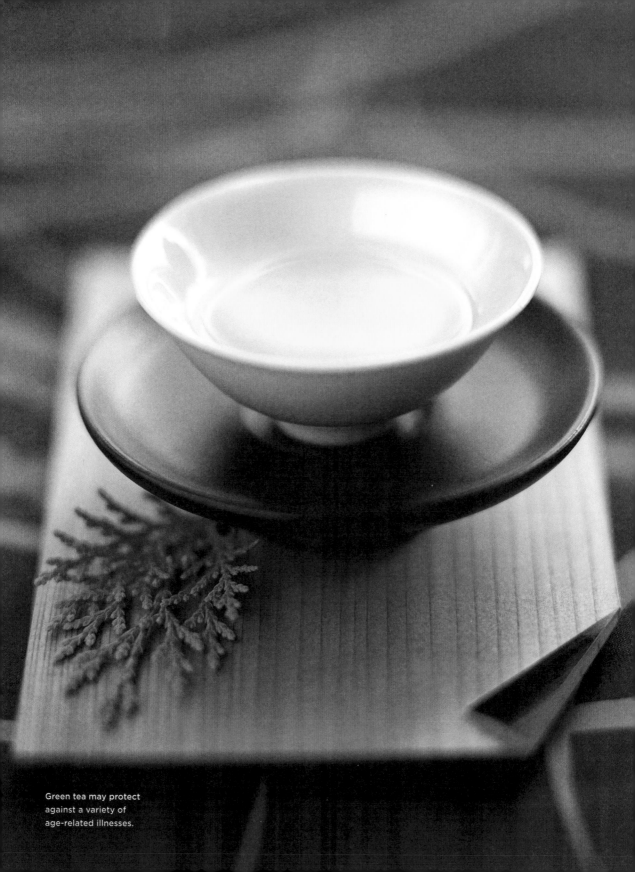

Green tea may protect
against a variety of
age-related illnesses.

# Top Longevity Hacks in Singapore

Singaporeans love plans. Sometimes it seems like they have a plan for everything. When it comes to living longer, the government's latest Healthy Living Master Plan includes a wide variety of creative "nudges" to improve everyday life for residents, who on average are living 20 years longer than they did in 1960. In fact, by 2030, one in five Singaporeans is expected to be age 65 or older. To carry out the plan, more than 20 government agencies have collaborated to make healthy living as natural and effortless as possible for everyone. Here are a few examples of popular outreach programs.

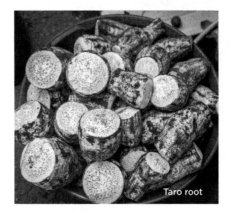
Taro root

**HEALTHY 365** | This mobility application uses games and rewards to encourage users to sign up for health challenges.

**I QUIT** | Due in part to this national 28-day anti-smoking campaign, the daily smoking rate in Singapore declined from 18 percent in 1992 to 14 percent in 2010, accounting for one of the lowest rates in the world.

**WOW** | Workplace Outreach Wellness (WOW) Package offers screenings for blood pressure, diabetes, and cholesterol; tips on weight management; and suggestions for healthy snacks to eat while at work.

**"HEALTHY CHOICE" LOGO** | Major supermarkets identify foods such as fruits and vegetables, whole grains, and lean proteins with a special label, offering some items at discounted prices.

**LET IT OUT** | Support groups such as Caregivers for Youth and CHAT Singapore offer tips and hotlines to aid teens and tweens dealing with pressures at school, heartache after a breakup, the loss of a loved one, or other situations.

**HEALTH AMBASSADORS** | Volunteers from all walks of life, including seniors, share information on subjects such as the importance of vaccinations or eating healthy foods.

**EAT, DRINK, SHOP HEALTHIER CHALLENGE** | Participants in this program earn redeemable "Healthpoints" for purchasing healthy meals, drinks, desserts, and groceries.

**HEALTHY WORKPLACE ECOSYSTEM** | Employers offer healthier food options, free exercise sessions, educational workshops, and health screenings to their workers.

**LOSE TO WIN** | Singapore's Health Promotion Board runs this 12-week national competition to lose weight through healthy lifestyle practices. In some contest seasons, participants have earned rewards for progress.

We strolled along a tree-lined walkway following the curve of the river. The waterfront here, once a center for shipping warehouses, had been converted into a kind of pedestrian mall with glitzy restaurants and nightclubs.

I asked Thong to meet me because I wanted to get her perspective on how Singapore had changed during the half century since she'd moved here from Malaysia. What did she think of life on the island today?

"My own life is very full," she said. Her family and volunteer work kept her busy. But she also did qigong for exercise, kept up with her yoga, and walked briskly when she could.

One of the groups she volunteered for was the Silver Generation Office, whose "ambassadors" knocked on the doors of elderly residents to make sure they're all right. I had to smile at the idea of her checking up on the "old folks."

"What about the government?" I asked. "Is it doing a good job?"

"I trust them," she said. "They've delivered what they've promised over the years, so when they ask people to get vaccinated or wear masks,

Billah Mustari, a neighborhood volunteer, tends the rooftop garden at the Khoo Teck Puat Hospital.

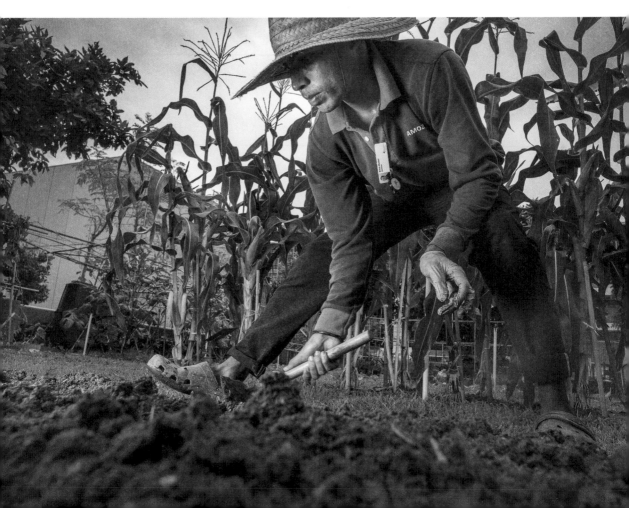

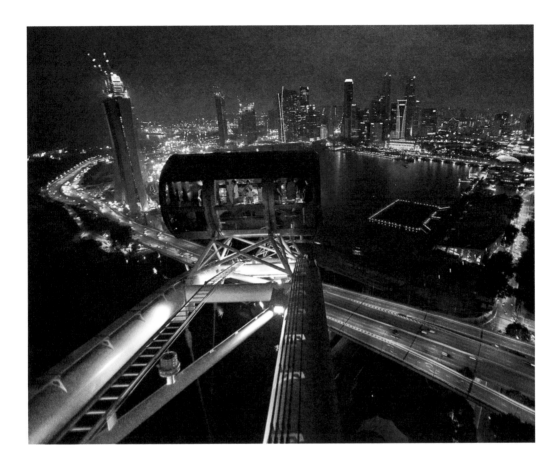

most everyone does. Besides, when the government makes a rule, it means business."

OK, that sounded tough but fair—a winning combination for Singapore's top-down approach to practically everything. What I wondered, then as now, was whether you could translate Singapore's public health successes into solutions for the United States, where trust in government was more elusive. Strategies designed for a society that valued consensus and security might not work in an argumentative, freedom-loving nation like our own, where issues tended to be settled through competition as much as cooperation.

In fact, that's the question on my mind every time I return from one of the world's blue zones, from Sardinia to Singapore, to focus on the lives of average Americans. Given all the challenges we face in this country, could we build health and longevity like theirs into our own communities, homes, and personal surroundings?

I'll spare you the suspense. The answer is yes.

Passengers inside the capsules of the Singapore Flyer, Asia's largest observation wheel, soar more than 500 feet above the city.

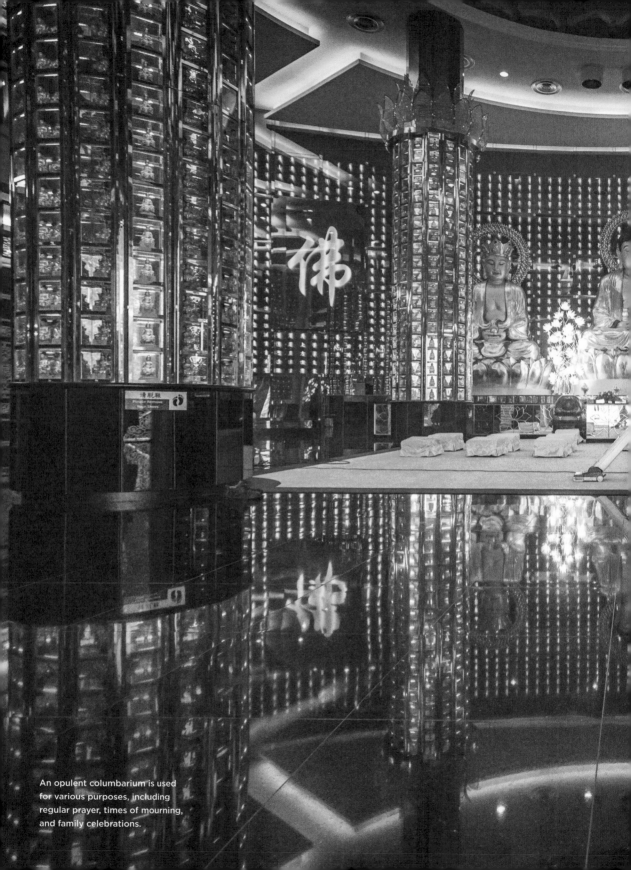

An opulent columbarium is used for various purposes, including regular prayer, times of mourning, and family celebrations.

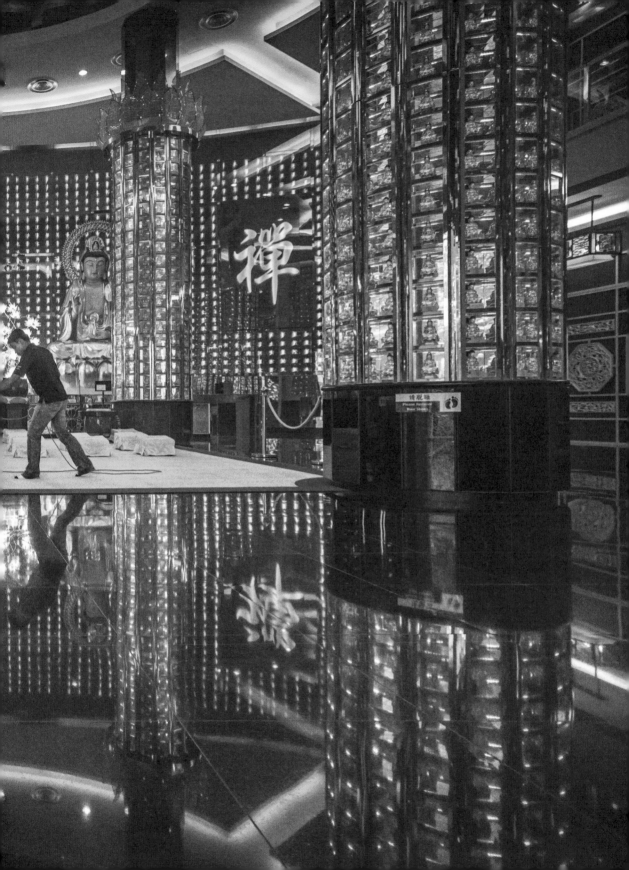

## LESSONS FROM SINGAPORE'S BLUE ZONE

■ **Choose a safe neighborhood in a safe city**
Pick a neighborhood with well-lit streets, free of graffiti. Join a neighborhood watch group and make it a point to know your neighbors at least three doors down on each side of your home.

■ **Live your values**
Take time to know your values and let them guide you in choosing a place to live, a social network, and a job. If your family is a priority, try to live near them. If you love to work with your hands, don't get a job in an office.

■ **Find your tribe**
Join a club, get involved at church, double down on your family, be the best sports fan you can. Likely you will feel more secure—and enjoy the camaraderie.

■ **Look for an environment of trust**
Move to a place where you trust your neighbors and local officials, work at a place where you trust your boss and co-workers, and seek out trustworthy friends. At a certain level, trust is more important than income.

■ **Buy good health care**
Make sure you're covered adequately by health insurance. It's hard to live happily if you're not healthy. Knowing that you'll get good care if you get sick removes one of the main stressors in life.

■ **Focus on financial success**
If status, financial security, and a sense of accomplishment are important to you, you might want to put most of your life's focus on making as much money as you can. For someone like you, by and large, the richer you get, the more satisfied you'll be.

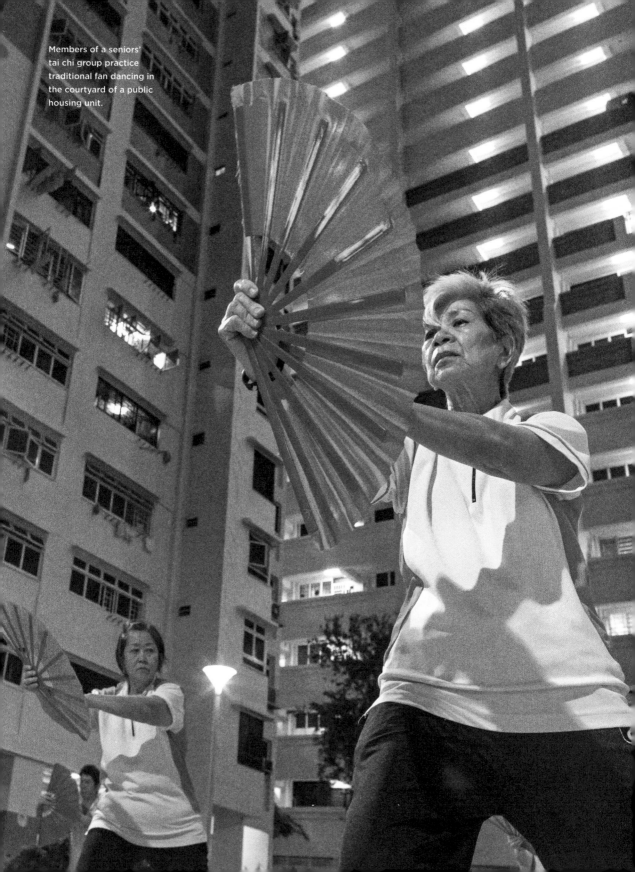

Members of a seniors' tai chi group practice traditional fan dancing in the courtyard of a public housing unit.

# PART II

# Building Your
# Blue Zone

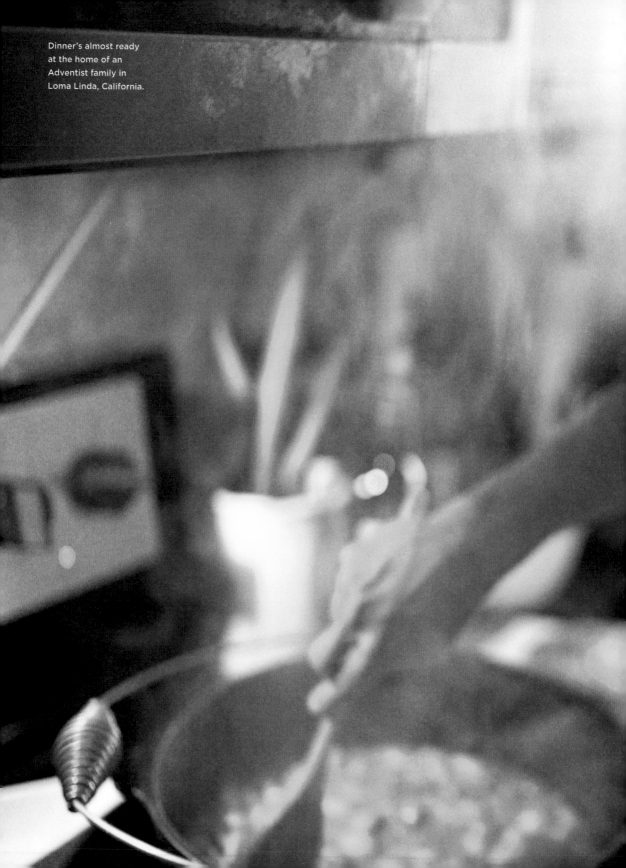

Dinner's almost ready
at the home of an
Adventist family in
Loma Linda, California.

# CHAPTER 7

# The Power 9

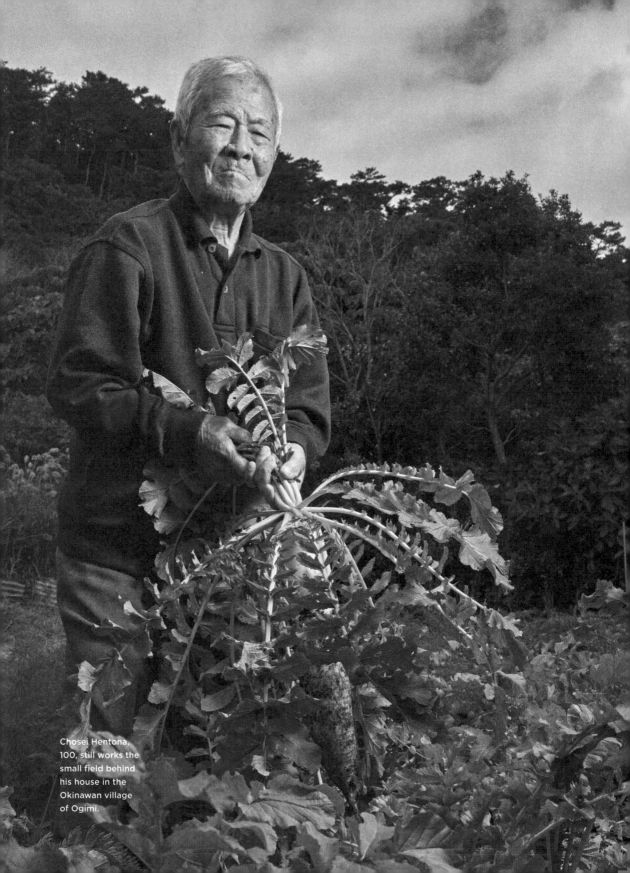

Chosei Hentona, 100, still works the small field behind his house in the Okinawan village of Ogimi.

# Rules to Live Longer By

The original idea behind Blue Zones was, in a sense, to reverse engineer longevity. Since only 20 percent or so of how long we live is dictated by our genes rather than our environment, I reasoned that if I could find the places where people lived the longest and discern the lifestyle factors common to all of them, I'd have something that resembled a formula for longevity.

Admittedly, I can't prove that the lifestyle factors I identified in each blue zone cause the extreme longevity of those who live there, but I do know they are highly correlated. And while several lifestyle characteristics are unique to each blue zone (such as bitter melon consumption in Okinawa and calcium-heavy water in Nicoya),

I found a remarkably consistent pattern in all blue zones. Correlation is not causation, but when you find the same longevity factors springing up independently in five vastly different cultures on four continents, you can't ignore it.

As I described in the previous chapters, I recruited teams of medical researchers, anthropologists, demographers, and epidemiologists to find the evidence-based commonalities among these remarkable places.

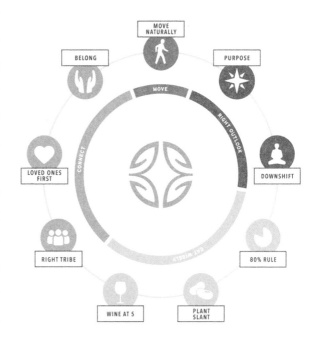

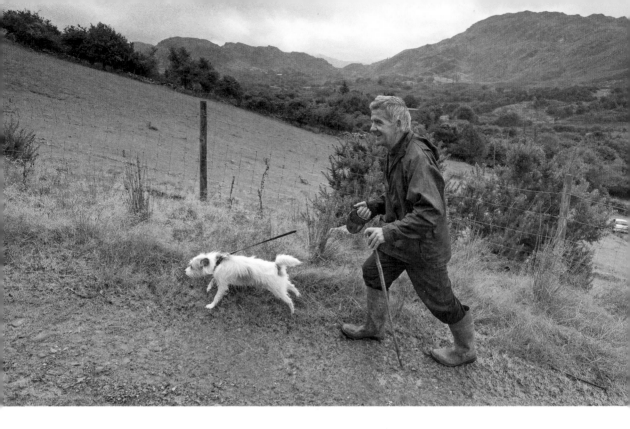

A man walks his dog on a drizzly country lane past farm fields in County Kerry, Ireland.

Together with local researchers who were studying centenarians, we cross-checked our working theories with academic papers and interviewed a representative sample of 90- and 100-year-olds in each blue zone. And what we discovered was that no one secret explained why these people tended to enjoy long, healthy lives. Instead, they benefited from an interconnected web of factors, including what they ate, their social networks, daily rituals, physical environments, and sense of purpose—all of which propelled them forward and gave their lives meaning.

In this chapter, we'll break down these factors into an action plan for you. As the Seventh-day Adventists have demonstrated, the average American's life expectancy could get a boost of seven to 10 years if he or she adopted a blue zones lifestyle. To show you how, we've distilled the world's best longevity practices into nine practical lessons to help you shape your surroundings for greater health and longer life. Think of it as a de facto formula for longevity—the best, most credible information available for adding years to your life and life to your years.

The secret to success, as you'll later discover, comes from creating an environment around yourself, your family, and your community that nudges you into the right behaviors subtly and relentlessly, just as the environments of the blue zones have done for the people who live in them. In Chapter 9, we'll show you how to do these things for long enough to actually add years to your life.

We designed the Power 9 to cover the following life domains: how to optimize your environment for a more active lifestyle; how to adopt the right outlook; how to eat wisely; and how to build social relationships that support your good habits.

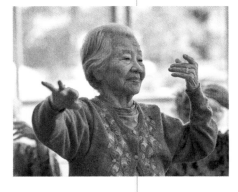

# ❶ Move Naturally

The world's longevity all-stars don't pump iron, run marathons, or join gyms. Instead, they live in environments that constantly nudge them into moving without thinking about it. By one estimate, people in the blue zones engage in some form of physical activity—gardening, food preparation, cleaning, or walking—every 10 to 15 minutes. Their streets are built for humans, not cars. Going to a friend's house, out to eat, to work, or to church is an opportunity for a walk.

At the community center in Ogimi, elderly women get together regularly to move to traditional music.

In Nicoya, women still grind corn and pat tortillas by hand. In Ikaria, they knead bread. In Okinawa, houses are almost devoid of furniture, so Okinawans get up and down from the floor dozens of times every day—even into their 90s and 100s.

WHAT TO DO:

Walking is one of the safest, easiest, and cheapest ways to move naturally throughout the day. Just walking 30 minutes a day can have a big impact on your health and mood. It can not only help prevent heart disease, depression,

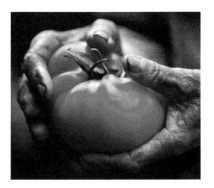

### GOZEI SHINZATO

Barely four and half feet tall, the 104-year-old Okinawan possessed the frenetic energy of a Chihuahua and the flexibility of a yogi. Just outside her three-room house in northern Okinawa, she kept a tidy garden filled with nutrient-rich, longevity-promoting foods, from sweet potatoes and soybeans to mugwort and turmeric. She tended her garden with a three-pronged hoe, working her way up and down the rows, or kneeling on a rubber pad to yank out weeds. Such regular, low-key physical activity not only reduces stress, experts say, but it also extends lifespans.

and obesity; it can also help you see your neighborhood, town, and city in a new way, explore local parks and trails safely, and make new friends and community connections.

Start by putting your walking or running shoes out where you can see them. (If you don't have running shoes or a bike, consider investing in them.)

Walking with a buddy or a group is even better. Research published in the *American Journal of Preventive Medicine* shows that people are more likely to walk for recreation or exercise when they are in the company of others or with their pet. Walking and talking is a way to connect while reaping the benefits of moving.

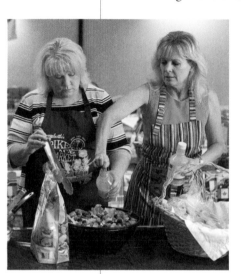

Adventist women put the finishing touches on dishes for a potluck meal at their church.

Scout out walking routes in your neighborhood. Draw a map of your neighborhood with the streets, parks, cafés, homes of people you know, landmark buildings, places to go, and anything else important that you might want to walk to. The goal is to meet and walk at least once per week (but more often is better).

You might also plan a walking meeting at work. It can be a great way to keep you and your co-workers more active—and when weather permits, getting some sunshine and fresh air helps relieve stress. Some workplaces have created walking paths on company grounds or walking-route maps to the neighborhoods around their office buildings. A recent survey by *Harvard Business Review* shows that teams who walk in groups say they are more creative. Bringing a group of co-workers together can also engage employees who otherwise might not get involved. In one study done by Wellness & Prevention, Inc., at Johnson & Johnson, groups that had walking meetings reported feeling more energized and more invested in their colleagues and organization. Management and employee barriers can also be lowered during a walking meeting.

Take the bus or public transportation to work or to run an errand. American Heart Association research has found that people who regularly take public transit are 44 percent less likely to be overweight, 27 percent less likely to have high blood pressure, and 34 percent less likely to have diabetes, compared with people who drive.

At home, set up a corner or other place with pillows where you can sit, read, or do work on the floor. Sitting on the floor works your thighs, glutes, and lower back each time you sit down and stand back up. Supporting yourself without a chairback improves posture and may help you burn up to an additional 130 calories each hour. If it's hard for you to go all the way down at first, you can transition by sitting on a medicine ball or a floor chair with a back until your muscles strengthen up.

# ❷ Purpose

People in the blue zones don't wake up feeling rudderless. They're invested in family, keeping their minds engaged, and keeping daily rituals to downshift and reduce stress. They're driven by their lives' meaning and purpose.

The Nicoyans called it *plan de vida,* and the Okinawans called it *ikigai:* For both, it translates to "why I wake up in the morning."

Research shows that a strong sense of purpose may reduce the chances of suffering from Alzheimer's disease, arthritis, and stroke. A National Institutes of Health–funded study looked at the correlation between having a sense of purpose and longevity. It found that healthy people between the ages of 65 and 92 who expressed having clear goals or a purpose lived up to seven years longer and were sharper than those who did not. This is because individuals who understand what brings them joy and happiness tend to have what we like to call the right outlook. They are engulfed in activities and communities that allow them to immerse themselves in a rewarding and gratifying environment.

For many people today, finding a sense of purpose may not be so easy. Your life might feel busier than ever,

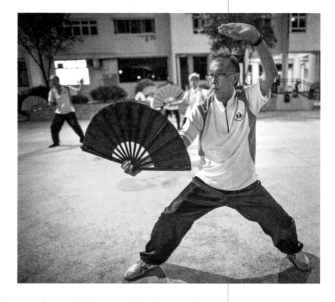

An exercise club practices a traditional fan dance outside a housing complex in Singapore.

whether you're chasing after a toddler, juggling childcare with a demanding job, putting in extra hours to finish a project, going back to school to learn a new skill, working two jobs to make ends meet, managing an illness, or caring for an elderly parent. When you find yourself racing from one task to the next from the moment you get up in the morning to the hour you fall into bed, there's precious little time to reflect on the meaning of it all.

But every now and then, you may catch yourself staring into the mirror, wondering if this is the life you really wanted—if this is what you were meant to do. At such a moment, ask yourself about your personal sense of purpose—your plan de vida, your ikigai—your reason for living besides work.

**WHAT TO DO:**

Write a purpose statement. Begin by answering the following questions developed by Dr. Richard Leider, author of *The Power of Purpose*:

Think about this sentence for a moment: "From family and friends who knew me when I was very young, I have heard that my 'special gifts' are _____." How have these "gifts" persisted in your life?

Imagine being on your deathbed, still clear and coherent, when your best friend drops in to visit you. Your friend asks, "Did you give and receive love?" "Were you authentically you?" "Did you make a small difference in the world?" How would you answer the questions?

Get out your calculator and do some "life math." Multiply your age times 365: _____. Then subtract that number from 30,000, an average life expectancy.

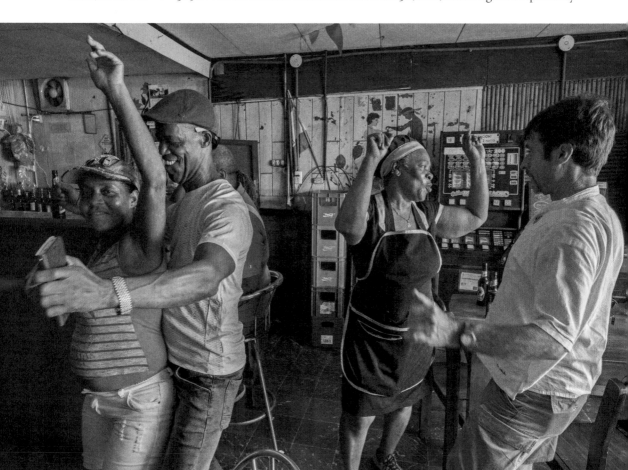

Divide that number by 365. Once you get clear that you have _____ more years to wake up, it might inspire you to live more courageously now. How do you feel about how you are spending your most precious currency—your time?

How did you wake up this morning? Did you resist getting up, or did you get out of bed with energy and purpose? Think about the way you wake up these days, and you will learn something about your life's purpose. What is your "mood" when you get up most days?

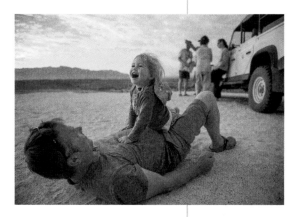

A young adventurer climbs on his dad during a rest stop in the Namibian desert.

Write the question "What are my gifts?" on five index cards. Give a card to five people who know you well and ask them to write their response to the question on the card. Put the cards all together in a place where you can see them. What theme or thread do you find?

Are you curious? What are you most curious about these days? Here are some clues that will help you answer: Time passes quickly when you're exploring this. It's so interesting, you can't help spending time on it! A bad day doing this is better than a good day doing most other things.

Look around you for potential models and mentors. Ask yourself who is really leading the kind of life and doing the kind of work that you envision in the next phase of your life. Initiate a courageous conversation to find out: What do they like most and least about their work?

## ❸ Downshift

Even people in the blue zones experience stress. But what the world's longest-lived people have that we don't are routines to shed that stress. Okinawans take a few moments each day to remember their ancestors, Adventists pray, Ikarians take a nap, and Sardinians do happy hour. Costa Ricans have a knack for creating happy moments every day, with no need for special occasions. Friends get together to watch soccer, play music, prepare carne asada (barbecue) with family or neighbors, drink beer, and tell lots of jokes.

"You walk around Costa Rica and everybody is saying *pura vida,*" said Carol Graham, an economist at the Brookings Institution who grew up in Latin America. Literally the phrase means "pure life," but it's commonly used to say "all good" and "take it easy."

For the Adventists in Loma Linda, California, the Saturday Sabbath represents a "sanctuary in time." From sunset Friday to sunset Saturday, they focus on God, their families, and nature. They don't work. Kids don't play organized sports or do homework. Instead, families do things together, such as hiking, that bring them closer to one another and to God. It's a time to put the rest of the week in perspective and to lessen the din and confusion of everyday life.

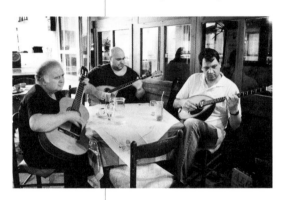

Musicians strike up a tune at an eating establishment on the Greek island of Ikaria.

Unlike many Americans, for whom accomplishment, status, and material wealth are highly revered, people in the blue zones don't get into the trap of overworking, over-spending, and undersocializing.

**WHAT TO DO:**

Start a meditation practice. There are many different ways to do it. They all typically involve a quiet, comfortable place to relax; a comfortable position (either sitting or lying down) that promotes meditation; focused attention; and letting distractions go as they come up. There are forms of "walking meditation" as well, but they have not been studied as thoroughly. Either way, setting aside as little as 15 minutes a day to "downshift" can benefit you in many ways.

Emotional benefits may include increased self-awareness, which may also help you find a purpose, or ikigai (another blue zones shared trait), reduce negative emotions that contribute to stress, develop skills to manage stress, increase creativity, and reduce symptoms of anxiety and depression. Since meditation has been shown to reverse the stress response, physical benefits include lowered blood pressure, reduced inflammation, support for smoking

**TAKE TIME TO UNPLUG**

"What are you standing out there for?" she asked. I had just hiked two hours through the tropical forest in Costa Rica and come upon her cottage. Her name was Segundia Zuniga, and she invited me in for coffee and cornbread. Her neighbors, a middle-age couple, were already inside, discussing the weather and the crops and indulging in a little harmless gossip. Her 91-year-old husband, Ildifonso, napped in a hammock. "Don't you ever get bored?" I asked. "What do you do to entertain yourself?" Not skipping a beat, she said, "I find a patch of shade and eat an orange."

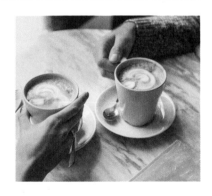

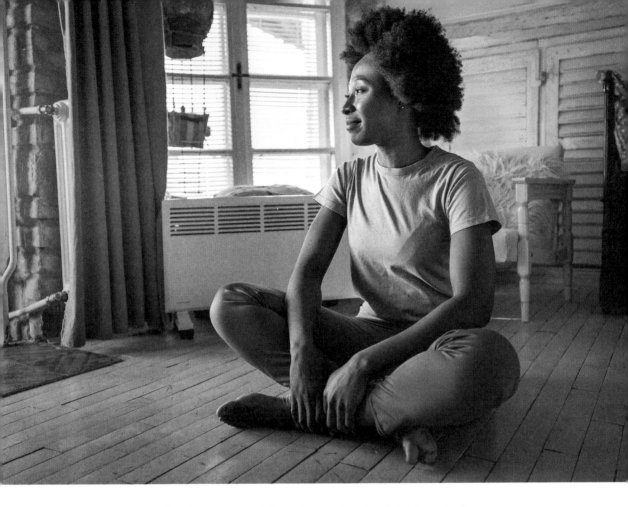

cessation programs, reduced symptoms of ulcerative colitis and irritable bowel syndrome, and treatment for chronic insomnia.

The CDC's National Health Interview Survey showed that meditation practice among adults tripled between 2012 and 2017.

One way to get started is to download a free meditation app or enroll in a series of meditation classes. Set up a meditation nook in a corner or room of your house. It should be a quiet place with a cushion you can sit on, decorated with the things that inspire you to downshift. Seeing this setup will be a visual reminder for you to meditate.

Another way to downshift: Watch a funny video on Facebook or YouTube. It can reduce stress as effectively as 20 minutes on a treadmill—and lift your spirits.

Limit your workweek to 40 hours and plan a vacation or time away from the workplace.

Write a thank-you note to a co-worker or friend. Research published in

One of many ways to "downshift" during a busy day, meditating also relieves stress.

*Psychological Science* says that when people express their gratitude, it improves both their own happiness and the well-being and happiness of the person they are thanking.

# ❹ 80 Percent Rule

If you've ever been lucky enough to eat with an Okinawan elder, you're likely to hear them intone these words at the start of a meal: *Hara hachi bu.*

"It's a Confucian-inspired adage," said Dr. Craig Willcox, co-author of *The Okinawa Program.* "All of the old folks say it before they eat. It means 'Eat until you are 80 percent full.'"

The idea behind the adage is that it takes about 20 minutes for the stomach to tell the brain it is full, he continued. "Undereating, as the theory goes, slows down the body's metabolism in a way such that it produces fewer damaging oxidants—agents that rust the body from within."

Unlike most Americans, who keep eating until their stomachs are full, traditional Okinawans stop as soon as they no longer feel hungry. This practice has another advantage. It provides a helpful nudge to stay fit. The 20 percent gap between not being hungry and feeling full could be the difference between losing weight and gaining it.

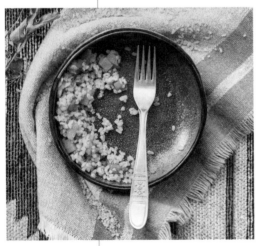

The Okinawan adage *Hara hachi bu* means to stop eating before one's stomach is full.

**WHAT TO DO:**

Eat more slowly. Eating faster results in eating more. Slow down to allow your body to respond to cues, which tell us we are no longer hungry. Focus on your food. Turn off the TV and the computer and phone. If you're going to eat, just eat. You'll eat more slowly, consume less, and savor the food more. Use smaller vessels. Choose to eat on smaller plates, and use tall, narrow glasses for drinks. You're likely to consume significantly less without even thinking about it.

Don't eat on the run. Instead of grabbing something to consume in the car, or while standing in front of the refrigerator, or while walking to your next meeting, sit down at a table. Make it a habit to eat purposefully, and you're more likely to appreciate the tastes and textures of your food.

Eat early in the day. In the blue zones, the biggest meal of the day is typically

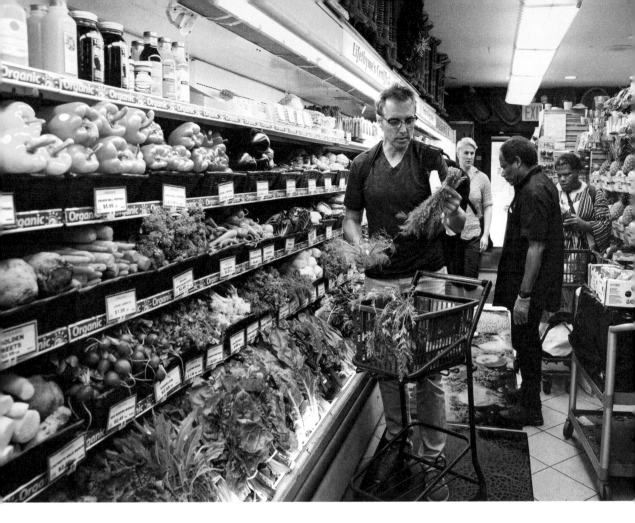

Dan grabs a bunch of healthy greens in the produce aisle at a vegan market in Manhattan.

eaten during the first half of the day. Nicoyans, Okinawans, and Sardinians eat their biggest meal at midday, while Adventists consume many of their calories for breakfast. All blue zones residents eat their smallest meal of the day late in the afternoon or early evening.

## ❺ Plant Slant

Until the late 20th century, the diets of every blue zone consisted almost entirely of minimally processed plant-based foods—mostly whole grains, greens, nuts, tubers, and beans. People ate meat—mainly pork—on average only five times a month. Serving sizes were three to four ounces, about the size of a deck of cards. Beans—including fava, black, and soy—and lentils were the true cornerstone of most centenarian diets.

Okinawans eat tofu every day, twice as much as people in the rest of Japan. Tofu is made from soybeans that are ground, boiled, strained, and then pressed into shapes. It's low in fat and high in protein and calcium, and some studies show it can lower cholesterol and the risk of prostate and breast cancer. Most towns on the island have shops where tofu is handmade. It's often still warm when it is sold, since it's delivered several times a day to grocery stores and markets all over the island.

Research from Harvard and an international group of scientists shows overwhelmingly that the closer you can get to eating this way, the less likely you will be to develop heart disease, diabetes, dementia, and several types of cancer.

**WHAT TO DO:**

Eat four to six vegetable servings a day. Blue zones diets always include at least two vegetables at each meal.

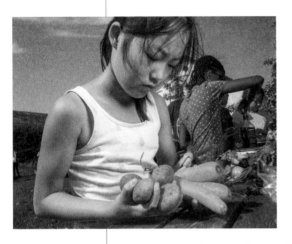

Schoolchildren in Denmark harvest vegetables they raised themselves as part of an environmental project.

Showcase fruits and vegetables in your kitchen. Put a beautiful bowl of fruit on the counter or table. At the bottom of it, leave a note that reads, "Fill me." Instead of hiding vegetables in the refrigerator compartment labeled "Produce," put them front and center on the shelves where you can see them.

Lead with beans. Make beans—or tofu—the centerpiece of lunches and dinners.

Eat nuts every day. The Adventist Health Studies show that it doesn't matter what kind of nuts you eat to help extend your life expectancy. But take note: A one-ounce serving of nuts typically ranges from 165 to 200 calories, so two ounces could be almost 400 calories.

Keep nuts available in your home, ideally in packages of two ounces or less. You might want to store them in the refrigerator to keep the oils fresh. Or keep a can of nuts in the office for an afternoon snack, which may help you avoid snacking right before dinner.

Limit your intake of meat. To emulate the blue zones diet, try to limit serving meat to twice weekly and serve no portions larger than a deck of cards.

## ❻ Wine@5

People in the blue zones (except Adventists) drink alcohol moderately and regularly. Moderate drinkers outlive nondrinkers. The trick is to drink one to two glasses per day (preferably Sardinian Cannonau wine), with friends and/or with food. And no, you can't save up all week and have 14 drinks on Saturday.

Epidemiological studies seem to show that people who have a daily drink of beer, wine, or spirits may accrue some health benefits. But the secrets of the blue zones suggest that consistency and moderation are key. In Okinawa, it's a daily glass of sake with friends. In Sardinia, it's a glass of dark red wine with each meal and whenever friends meet.

Red wine offers an extra bonus in that it contains artery-scrubbing polyphenols that may help fight arteriosclerosis. But beware the toxic effects of alcohol on the liver, brain, and other organs—along with an increased risk of accidents—when daily consumption exceeds a glass or two.

### WHAT TO DO:

Buy a case of high-quality red wine. The Sardinians quaff Cannonau in their blue zone, which you can find online by googling "Blue Zones wine." Dr. Christina Chrysohoou and colleagues found that a glass of wine with a plant-based meal actually increases antioxidant absorption.

Treat yourself to a happy hour. Set up yours to include a glass of wine, nuts as an appetizer, and a gathering of friends or time with a spouse.

A group of Sardinian friends toast one another, saying, *"A kent'annos* —May you live to be 100."

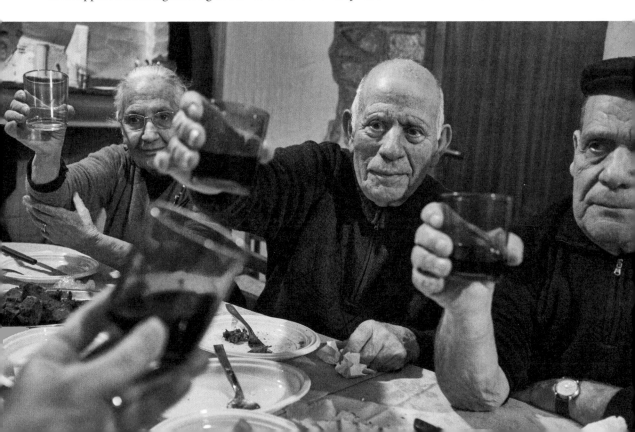

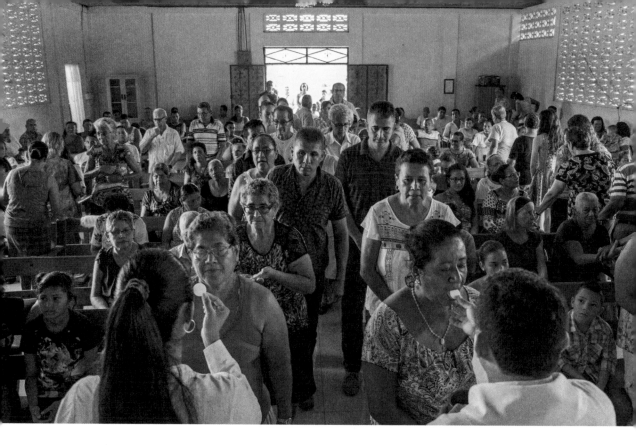

Parishioners take Communion during mass in a small church on Costa Rica's Nicoya Peninsula.

Take it easy. A serving or two per day of red wine is the most you need to drink to take advantage of its health benefits. Overdoing it negates any benefits you might enjoy, so drink in moderation.

# ❼ Belong

Healthy centenarians everywhere have faith. All but a handful of the centenarians we've interviewed belonged to a faith-based community. The Sardinians and Nicoyans are mostly Catholic. Okinawans have a blended religion that stresses ancestor worship. Loma Linda centenarians are Seventh-day Adventists. Denomination doesn't seem to matter. The simple act of worship is one of those subtly powerful habits that seems to improve your chances of having more good years. Research shows that attending faith-based services four times per month will add four to 14 years of life expectancy.

**WHAT TO DO:**

Be more involved. If you already belong to a religious community, take a more active role in the organization. The longevity-enhancing effect may be a function of how you attend rather than the fact you just attend. Get involved in an activity such as singing in the choir or volunteering, and it might enhance your well-being and extend your life.

Explore a new tradition. If you don't belong or have drifted away from the faith community of your birth, try to find a new one that matches your current values and worldview. Start by asking friends or people you admire to make some suggestions. If you are not sure, attend services in a different location once a week for the next eight weeks.

Just go. Schedule an hour a week for the next eight weeks (the time it takes to form a habit) to attend religious services. Don't think about it. Just go and do so with an open mind. Studies show that people who get involved with the service (singing hymns, participating in prayers or liturgy, volunteering) may find their well-being enhanced.

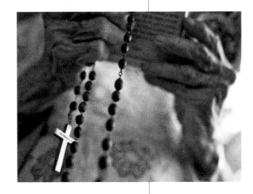

Faith and prayer are thought to be significant factors in extending longevity.

## ❽ Loved Ones First

Successful centenarians in the blue zones put their families first. This means keeping aging parents and grandparents nearby or in the home. (It lowers disease and mortality rates of children in the home, too.) They commit to a life partner (which can add up to three years of life expectancy) and invest in their children with time and love (and who will be more likely to care for you when the time comes).

In Nicoya, families tend to live in clusters. In one village I visited, all 99 inhabitants were descended from the same 85-year-old man. They still met for meals at a family-owned restaurant, and the patriarch's grandchildren still

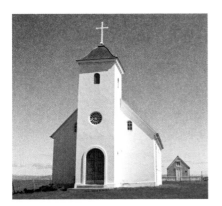

### THE SCIENCE BEHIND BELONGING

Robert A. Hummer and a research team at the University of Texas found that people who never went to church had a 1.87 times higher risk of death in their study's nine-year follow-up period than those who attended more than once a week. Their explanation: Going to church appeared to improve social ties, such as being married, keeping active, and having friends or relatives to call on; and encouraged healthy behaviors, such as avoiding smoking and drinking. Other research has found that women who frequently attended church had a 33 percent reduced chance of dying, compared with those who didn't.

visited him daily to help him tidy up or just to play a game of checkers.

In Sardinia, I once asked a vineyard owner who was caring for his infirm mother if it wouldn't be easier to put her in a home. He wagged his finger at me. "I wouldn't even think of such a thing. It would dishonor my family."

America is trending in the opposite direction. In many busy families with working parents and active kids, family time can become rare as everyone's schedules become more and more packed with things to do. How to buck the trend? Gail Hartman, a licensed psychologist, said the key was for all generations of a family to commit to spending time together. "Successful families make a point of eating at least one meal a day together, taking annual vacations, and spending family time. Everything does not need to stop. Kids can be doing homework, and parents can be preparing dinner, but the point is there is a 'we-ness' to the family."

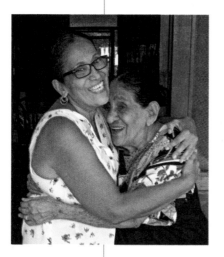

Natividad Talia Matarrita Fonseca, 93, gets a hug from her daughter Sara Fonseca at her home in Costa Rica.

**WHAT TO DO:**

Establish rituals. Children thrive on repetition. Make one family meal a day sacred. Establish a tradition for a family vacation. Have dinner with Grandma every Tuesday night. Make a point to purposefully celebrate holidays.

Create a family shrine. In Okinawan homes, the ancestor shrine is always displayed in the best room in the house. It showcases pictures of deceased loved ones and their important possessions. Try picking a wall to display pictures of your parents and children, or take annual family pictures and display them in progression.

Get closer. It's easier for families to bond and spend time together in a smaller space. A large, spread-out house makes it easier for family members to segment themselves from the group. If you live in a large home, establish one room where family members gather daily.

Put family first. Invest time and energy in your children, your spouse, and your parents. Play with your children, nurture your marriage, and honor your parents.

## ❾ Right Tribe

One of the most profound, measurable, and long-lasting things you can do to adopt a blue zones lifestyle is to build a social circle around yourself that supports healthy eating, activity, and emotional well-being.

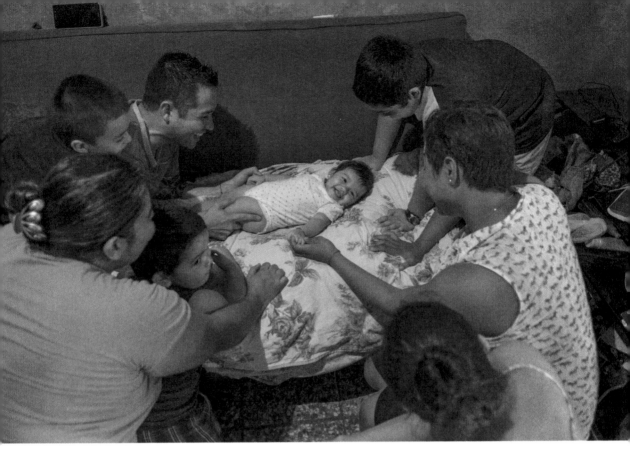

The world's longest-lived people chose—or were born into—social circles that encourage healthy behaviors. In Okinawa, children were traditionally put into *moais,* a lifelong circle of friends that supported individuals well into old age. One particular moai that I spent some time with was made up of a group of women whose average age was 102. They got together every evening to drink sake and socialize. Although the lifestyles of younger generations have changed in recent decades, some of the world's oldest women still live in Okinawa.

Research shows that friends and family can have a long-term impact on our health. The sort of people we hang out with has an enormous and measurable influence not only on how happy we are, but also on how fat or even how lonely we are. In fact, if your best friends don't live healthily, you likely don't either. You are the sum of the people you spend the most time with, so spend some time optimizing your social circle for better health and happiness.

Americans had an average of three close friends in the 1980s. Today that number has dropped to between one and two. If you don't have at least three friends you can call up on a bad day, research shows that you're shaving about eight years off your life expectancy.

A joyful family surrounds a five-month-old girl in Nicoya, Costa Rica, where support from loved ones is key to living longer.

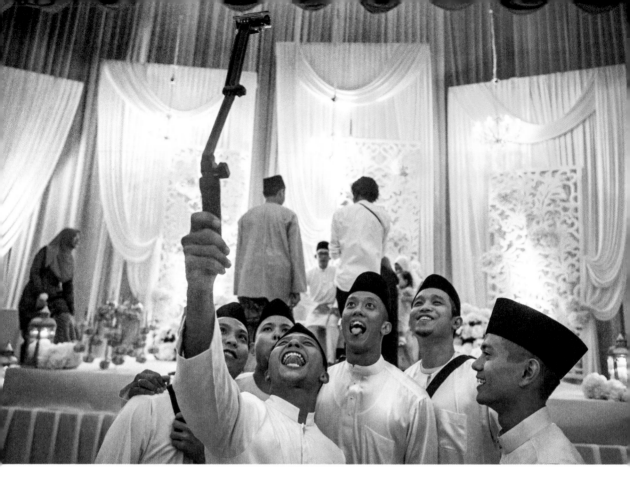

Young men mug for a selfie before the wedding of a Malay couple in Singapore.

Studies have found that happiness is contagious—as are smoking, obesity, and loneliness. The social circles of long-lived people have favorably shaped their health behaviors. To reap the benefits that blue zones residents experience, reach out more socially and nurture strong friendships. The more you socialize, the happier—and healthier—you'll be.

The most profound antidote to loneliness is through service. When we step out of our world and help others in need, we realize our value and build self-worth. It can be helping a neighbor who is struggling in isolation or collecting donations for a local shelter.

WHAT TO DO:

Volunteer. People who volunteer tend to lose weight, have lower rates of heart disease, and report higher levels of happiness. Volunteering also opens up opportunities to meet like-minded people with the same values. Decide what you do best and volunteer your time. Check out online sites such as VolunteerMatch. Call or email organizations that most interest you. Ask if they have an initiation period or some sort of training to see if it's the right fit for you. Ask about opportunities to socialize or connect with other volunteers. This could be a good place for you to build your social circle with like-minded people. Ask how the organization recognizes volunteers. The best ones have volunteer socials or recognition events. If you don't have a positive experience the first time you go, then you won't want to go back. Remember: For it to be sustainable, it must be an experience that you like.

Join a new social group. This might be a new group at your temple, church, or other faith-based community; a new club at your school; or a local group like those found on Meetup.

Start a moai: Invite four to eight people to join your group. Select an activity such as walking or sharing a potluck meal or happy hour. Pick a start date and a day and time to meet at least once a week (twice a week or more is better). Set up a way to stay in touch regularly, even outside your meetups, such as a group email, text chain, or closed Facebook group or within an app like WhatsApp so that your members can easily and regularly communicate. Choose routes, trails, or neighborhoods to walk in. Decide who will host the first potluck event and other future locations (parks, etc.).

Strengthen your friendships. Look around your existing social network to see if there is potential to deepen casual connections. If you're a parent, is there another parent you see at school drop-off who seems to have good energy? Or a co-worker you banter with? Chat them up. Ask them if they'd like to get coffee or lunch sometime. Ask for their phone number to finalize plans and keep in touch. Invite them to a casual gathering or outing with one or two other people.

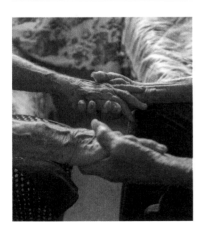

### RIGHT TRIBE

In his book *Together: The Healing Power of Human Connection in a Sometimes Lonely World*, former surgeon general Dr. Vivek Murthy makes the case that loneliness is a worldwide experience. In the United States, surveys indicate that at least 22 percent of adults struggle with loneliness, and many other countries have double-digit rates. Loneliness is as bad for health as smoking 15 cigarettes a day, potentially leading to conditions such as cancer, heart disease, or dementia. Combating loneliness begins with self-confidence, Murthy says. We may feel lonely because we think we're unlikable or not "good enough," a feeling made worse when we focus on everybody else's "perfect" lives on social media.

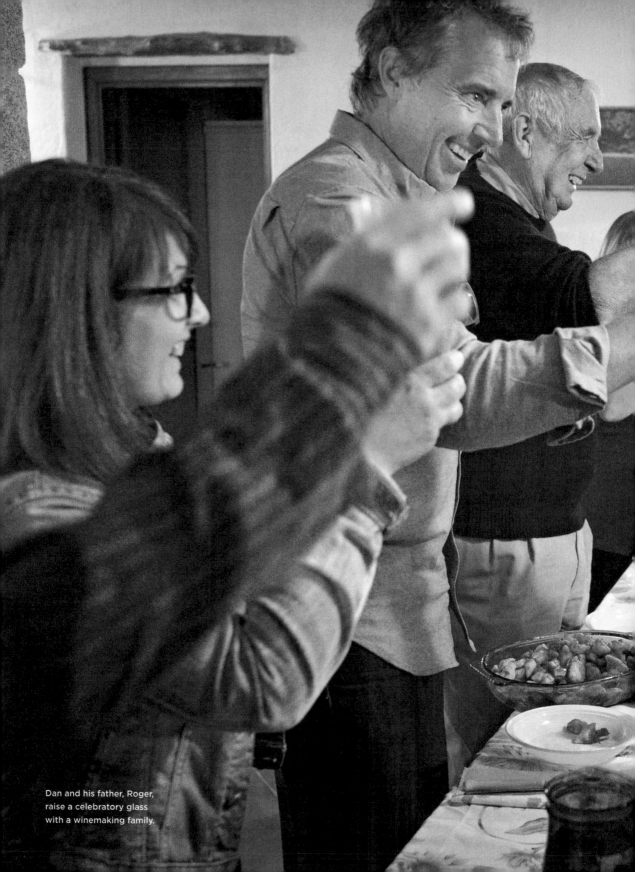

Dan and his father, Roger, raise a celebratory glass with a winemaking family.

# CHAPTER 8

# The Blue Zones Food Guidelines

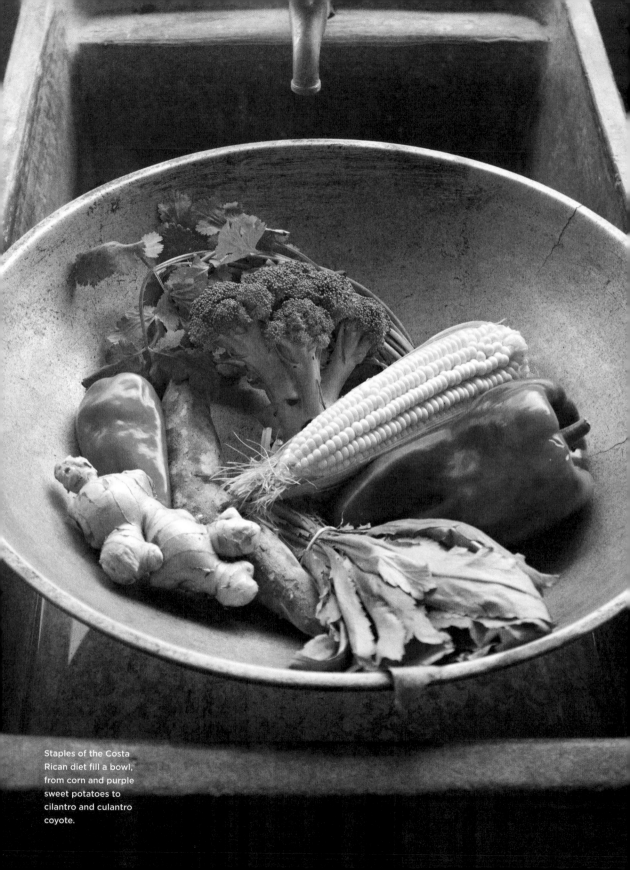

Staples of the Costa Rican diet fill a bowl, from corn and purple sweet potatoes to cilantro and culantro coyote.

# How to Eat Smarter

People in the blue zones don't just eat to live; they also live to eat, and they eat for enjoyment as much as anyone else. As we look for ways to adapt their foods and customs to fit our own lifestyles, the idea isn't to kill the pleasures of eating but to crowd out the junk food from our daily routine with foods the longest-lived people eat—and to enjoy doing it.

In many parts of the United States, people are still drowning in a sea of cheap calories that seems impossible to escape. You can't walk through an airport, pay cash for gasoline, or buy cough medicine without being confronted by a barrage of salty snacks, candy bars, and sodas. Restaurant food portions—mostly meaty and cheesy—have grown supersized. And the processed food and beverage industry hires the sharpest minds on Madison Avenue and spends more than $10 billion a year to convince us to eat food that erodes our health.

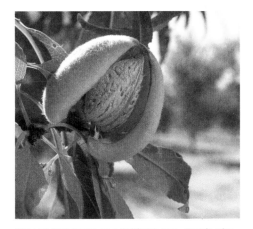

Almond fruit ripens on a California tree. People who eat nuts daily outlive those who don't by at least two years.

Too often we overeat. The average American woman consumes about 2,500 calories daily, and the average American man consumes about 3,200 calories. People in the blue zones eat about 20 percent less on average. In other words, 2,000 calories for a woman and 2,560 calories for a man. The goal is to feed your body in the best way possible.

The ideas in this chapter will help you do that. We've distilled more than 150 dietary surveys of the world's longest-lived peoples to tease out the secrets of their food regimens. Blue zones inhabitants live longer because they've eaten the right foods—and avoided the wrong ones—for most of their lives. They've eaten this way not because they possessed heroic discipline, but because the healthiest foods were the cheapest and most accessible to them. Their kitchens were set up so that it was easy to make these foods. They spent time with people who ate the same way. And they possessed time-honored recipes to make healthy food taste good. To encourage you to do the same, we've simplified the diets of the world's longest-lived populations into 11 simple guidelines for your own longevity food regimen.

## Aim for at least a 95 percent plant-based diet

People in the blue zones consume an impressive variety of garden vegetables in season, and then they pickle or dry the surplus to enjoy during the off-season. The best-of-the-best longevity foods are leafy greens such as spinach, kale, beet and turnip tops, chard, and collards. Combined with seasonal fruits and veg-

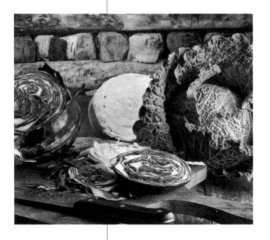

etables, whole grains, and beans, they dominate blue zones meals all year long.

Increasing the amount of plant-based foods in your meals can have many salutary effects. Beans, greens, yams and sweet potatoes, fruits, nuts, and seeds should all be favored. Whole grains are OK, too. Try a variety of fruits and vegetables, know which ones you like, and keep your kitchen stocked with them.

Many oils derive from plants, and they are all preferable to animal-based fats. We cannot say that olive oil is the only healthy plant-based oil, but it is the one most often used in the blue zones. Evidence shows that olive oil consumption increases good cholesterol and lowers bad cholesterol. In Ikaria, we found that for middle-age people, about six tablespoons of olive oil daily seemed to cut the risk of dying in half.

Adding cabbage to your diet, whether it's red, white, or the savoy variety, also adds antioxidants and other nutrients.

HOW TO DO IT:

- Keep favorite fruits and vegetables on hand. If you don't have access to fresh, affordable vegetables, frozen veggies are just fine.
- Use olive oil instead of butter. Drizzle it over steamed or boiled vegetables.

- Stock up on whole grains like oats, barley, brown rice, and ground corn. Grains used in the blue zones contain less gluten than modern wheat strains.
- Use leftover veggies to make vegetable soup or freeze them to serve later.

## Retreat from meat

People in four of the five original blue zones consumed meat, but they did so sparingly, using it as a celebratory food, a small side, or a way to flavor dishes. Averaging out consumption in blue zones, we found that people ate about two ounces or less of meat about five times per month. And we don't know if they lived longer despite eating meat.

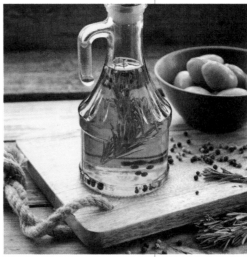

Extra-virgin olive oil, especially when drizzled unheated over food, may help protect against heart disease.

The Adventist Health Study-2, which has been following 96,000 Americans since 2002, has found that the people who live the longest are vegans or pesco-vegetarians, who eat a plant-based diet that includes a small amount of fish. Okinawans probably offer the best meat substitute: extra-firm tofu, which is high in protein and cancer-fighting phytoestrogens.

Research suggests that the closer you can get to a whole-food, plant-based diet, the less likely you are to develop heart disease, dementia, diabetes, and several types of cancer. Thirty-year-old vegetarian Adventists will likely outlive their meat-eating counterparts by as many as eight years. Since high-fat foods such as animal products and snack foods napalm your taste buds, you'll find that without meat, you'll enjoy the subtle flavors and textures that plant-based foods provide even more.

HOW TO DO IT:

- Avoid bringing beef, hot dogs, luncheon meats, or sausages into your house.
- If you must eat meat, reserve it for special occasions.
- Choose restaurants that offer delicious plant-based offerings. Thai, Indian, and Mexican restaurants almost always have plant-based options.

## Go easy on fish

In most blue zones, people ate some fish, but less than you might think—up to three small servings a week. In most cases, the fish being eaten were small and

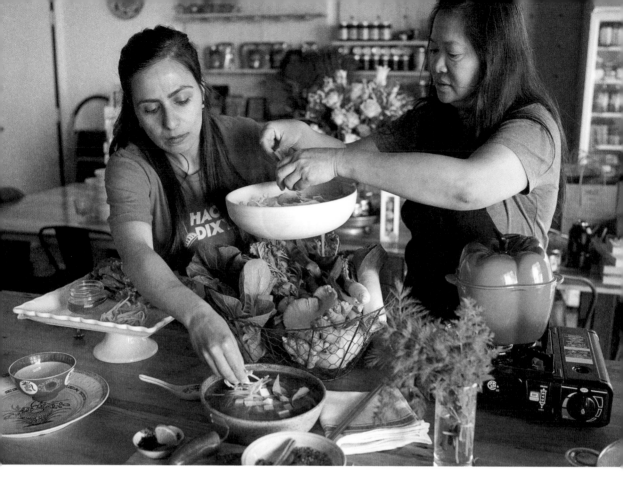

Dixya Bhattarai, a dietician, and Hao Tran, a science teacher, teamed up to open a healthy food restaurant and market in Fort Worth, Texas.

relatively inexpensive, such as sardines and anchovies—middle-of-the-food-chain species not exposed to the high levels of mercury or other chemicals like PCBs that pollute the gourmet fish supply today. If you must eat fish, eat fewer than three ounces up to three times weekly.

HOW TO DO IT:

- Learn what three ounces looks like, whether it's larger fish such as snapper and trout or smaller fish such as sardines and anchovies.
- Avoid predator fish such as swordfish, shark, and tuna. Avoid overfished species such as Chilean sea bass.
- Steer clear of farmed fish, as they are typically raised in overcrowded pens that make it necessary to use antibiotics, pesticides, and coloring.

## Reduce dairy

Milk from cows doesn't figure significantly in any blue zones diet except that of some Adventists. Arguments against milk often focus on its high fat and sugar content. Neal Barnard, the founder and president of the Physicians Committee for Responsible Medicine, points out that 49 percent of the calories in whole milk and about 70 percent of the calories in cheese come from fat—and that much of this fat is saturated. About 55 percent of the calories in skim milk come from lactose sugar. The number of people who (often unknowingly) have some difficulty digesting lactose may be as high as 60 percent. Goat's and sheep's milk products figure into the Ikarian and Sardinian blue zones.

We don't know if it's the goat's milk or sheep's milk that makes people healthier, or if it's the fact that the people climb up and down the same hilly terrain as the goats do. Interestingly, though, most goat's milk is consumed not as liquid but fermented as yogurt, sour milk, or cheese. Although goat's milk contains lactose, it also contains lactase, an enzyme that helps the body digest lactose.

HOW TO DO IT:

- Try unsweetened soy, coconut, or almond milk as a dairy alternative. Most have as much protein as regular milk.
- Satisfy occasional cravings with cheese made from grass-fed goat's or sheep's milk. Try Sardinian pecorino sardo or Greek feta. Both are rich, so you need only a small amount to flavor food.
- Small amounts of sheep's milk or goat's milk products—especially full-fat, naturally fermented yogurt with no added sugars—may be OK.

## SOCIAL CIRCLE CHECKLIST

Healthy behaviors are as contagious as a cold. Here are some ways to make sure you're part of a social circle with the greatest longevity benefits:

- Do your friends smoke?
- Are they overweight because of bad health behavior?
- Do they drink more than two drinks a day?
- Do they favor junk food or whole food?
- Are they usually upbeat, or do they like to complain?
- Is their idea of having fun watching TV or doing something active outdoors?
- Are they curious about the world?
- Do you feel better when you're around them?

While we wouldn't tell you to drop your old friends, we might encourage you to spend more time with your healthier new ones.

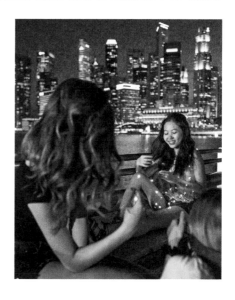

## Eliminate eggs

Though people in the blue zones eat some eggs, we don't recommend them. Consumption of eggs has been correlated to higher rates of prostate cancer for men and exacerbated kidney problems for women. Some people with heart or circulatory problems choose to forgo eggs. Again, eggs aren't necessary for living a long life. Moreover, people with diabetes should be cautious of eating egg yolks.

HOW TO DO IT:

- If you must buy eggs, buy only organic eggs from cage-free, pastured chickens.
- Substitute eggs with fruit or other plant-based foods such as whole-grain porridge or bread.
- When baking, you can use a quarter cup of applesauce, a quarter cup of mashed potatoes, or a small banana to substitute for one egg.

Many wild herbs such as myrtle, thyme, rosemary, helichrysum, and saffron have both culinary and medicinal uses.

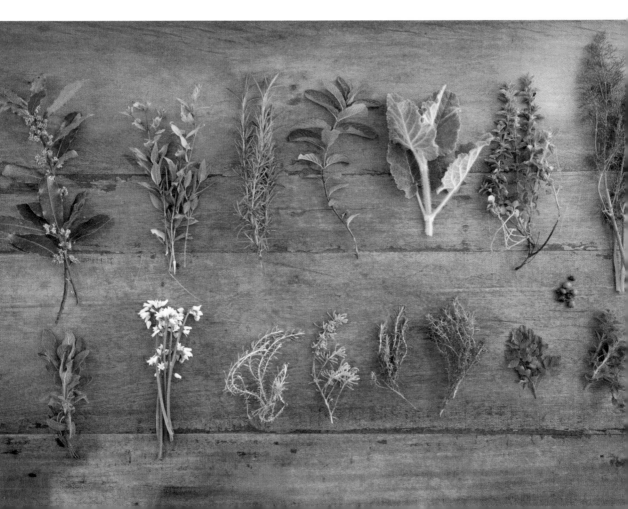

## Daily dose of beans

Beans reign supreme in the blue zones. People in these regions eat at least four times as many as Americans do on average. In Nicoya, it tends to be black beans. In the Mediterranean, they prefer lentils, garbanzo beans, and white beans. In Okinawa, people eat soybeans.

We recommend you consume at least one cup of cooked beans daily, because beans are the consummate superfood. On average, they are made up of 21 percent protein, 77 percent complex carbohydrates (the kind that deliver a slow and steady energy rather than the spike you get from refined carbohydrates like white flour), and only a small percentage of fat. They are also an excellent source of fiber. They're cheap and versatile, come in a variety of textures, and are packed with more nutrients per gram than any other food on Earth. And because beans are so hearty and satisfying, they'll likely push less healthy foods out of your diet.

Black-eyed peas, onions, fennel, and tomatoes make this Ikarian stew one of Dan's favorites.

HOW TO DO IT:

- Keep a variety of beans in your pantry. Dry beans are cheapest, but canned beans are quicker.
- Learn how to make one bean dish you enjoy.
- Make salads heartier by sprinkling cooked beans over them. Serve hummus or black bean cakes with salad.

## Slash sugar

Between 1970 and 2000, the amount of added sugar in the American food supply rose by 25 percent. This adds up to about 22 teaspoons of added sugar for each of us daily—insidious, hidden sugars mixed into soda, yogurt, and sauces. Too much sugar in our diet has been shown to suppress the immune system. It also spikes insulin levels, which can lead to diabetes and lower fertility, as well as make you fat and even shorten your life.

People in the blue zones eat sugar intentionally, not by habit or accident. They consume about the same amount of naturally occurring sugars found in fruits, vegetables, and even milk as Americans do. But they eat only a fraction of the added sugar—no more than seven teaspoons a day.

Our advice: If you must eat sweets, save cookies, candy, and bakery items for special occasions, ideally as part of a meal. Limit the sugar added to coffee, tea, and other foods to no more than four teaspoons per day. Skip any product that lists sugar among its first five ingredients.

HOW TO DO IT:

- Make honey your go-to sweetener. It's harder to spoon in and doesn't dissolve in cold liquids, so you tend to consume less of it—and more intentionally.
- Avoid sugar-sweetened sodas, teas, or fruit drinks. Try seltzer instead.
- Limit desserts or treats to 100 calories. Eat one serving a day or less.
- Consider fruit your sweet treat.
- Watch out for processed foods with added sugar, particularly sauces, salad dressings, and ketchup.
- Watch out for low-fat products. Some low-fat yogurts contain more sugar per ounce than soft drinks.

## Snack on nuts

The Adventist Health Study-2 found that people who eat nuts outlive those who don't by an average of two to three years. In Sardinia and Ikaria, they like almonds. In Nicoya, they prefer pistachios. The Adventists are keen on all kinds of nuts.

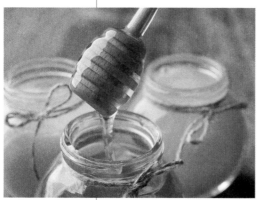

We recommend you eat two handfuls of nuts per day. The optimal mix: almonds (high in vitamin E and magnesium), peanuts (high in protein and folate, a B vitamin), Brazil nuts (high in selenium, a mineral found to be effective in protecting against prostate cancer), cashews (high in magnesium), and walnuts (high in alpha-linolenic acid, the only omega-3 fat found in a plant-based food). Walnuts, peanuts, and almonds are the nuts most likely to lower your cholesterol.

Besides sweetening coffee and tea, honey is also used in some blue zones to treat colds and even wounds.

HOW TO DO IT:

- Keep nuts around your workplace for midmorning or midafternoon snacks. Take small packages for travel and car trips.
- Try adding nuts or other seeds to salads and soups.
- Stock up on a variety of nuts, including almonds, peanuts, Brazil nuts, cashews, and walnuts.

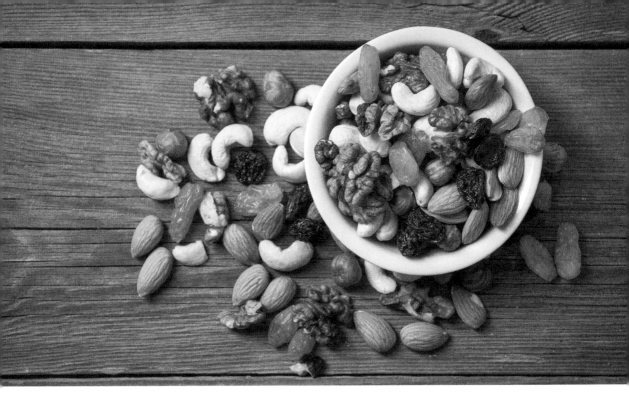

- Incorporate nuts into regular meals as a protein source.
- Eat some nuts before a meal to reduce the overall glycemic load.

Eating at least two handfuls of nuts a day can reduce "bad" LDL cholesterol by 9 to 20 percent.

## Sour on bread

Blue zones bread is unlike what most Americans buy. Commercially available breads often start with bleached white flour, which metabolizes quickly into sugar and spikes insulin levels. But bread from the blue zones is either whole grain or sourdough, each with its own healthful characteristics.

In Ikaria and Sardinia, breads are made from a variety of whole grains, including wheat, rye, and barley, each of which offers a wide spectrum of nutrients, such as tryptophan, an amino acid, and the minerals selenium and magnesium. Whole grains also have higher levels of fiber than most commonly used wheat flours.

Some traditional blue zones breads are made with naturally occurring bacteria called lactobacilli, which "digest" the starches and glutens while making the bread rise. The process also creates an acid—the "sour" in sourdough. The result is bread with even less gluten than breads labeled "gluten free," and with a longer shelf life than other types of breads and a pleasantly sour taste that most people like. Traditional sourdough breads actually lower the glycemic load of meals, making your entire meal healthier, slower burning, more digestible,

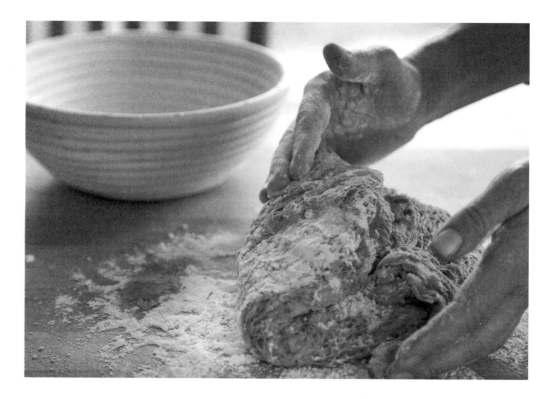

easier on your pancreas, and more likely to use calories as energy rather than store calories as fat.

We recommend you eat only sourdough or whole-grain breads.

**HOW TO DO IT:**

- Make sourdough bread yourself. Ed Wood, a fellow *National Geographic* writer, offers advice on sourdough starters at sourdo.com.
- Try sprouted-grain bread—among the most nutritious of foods.
- Choose whole-grain rye or pumpernickel bread over whole wheat. Look for bread that lists rye flour as the first ingredient. Most supermarket breads aren't true rye breads.
- In general, if you can squeeze a slice of bread into a ball, avoid it.

## Go wholly whole

A good definition of a "whole food" is one that is made of a single ingredient, raw, cooked, ground, or fermented, and not highly processed. Tofu is minimally processed, for example, while cheese-flavored corn puffs are highly processed.

People in the blue zones eat whole foods. They don't throw the yolk away to make an egg-white omelet, or spin the fat out of their yogurt, or juice the fiber-rich pulp out of their fruits. They also don't enrich or add extra ingredients to change the nutritional profile of their foods. Instead of taking vitamins or other supplements, they get everything they need from nutrient-dense, fiber-rich whole foods.

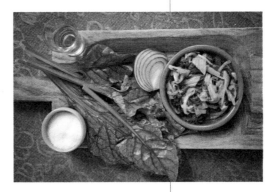

Blue zones dishes typically consist of a half dozen or so ingredients. Almost all the foods consumed by centenarians in the blue zones grow within a 10-mile radius of their homes. They eat raw fruits and vegetables; they grind whole grains themselves and then cook them slowly. They use fermentation—an ancient way to make nutrients bioavailable—in the tofu, sourdough bread, wine, and pickled vegetables they eat. And they rarely ingest artificial preservatives.

To make your meals wholly whole, try adding vegetables such as broccoli, cabbage, or cauliflower, which have been known to help protect the heart, stave off cancer, and lower oxidative stress. Finish dishes with olive oil. Supplement foods with herbs and spices. Don't forget to include beans for fiber. Finally, enjoy your meal with red wine.

Whether it's served in a salad or stew, Swiss chard offers an abundance of vitamins A, C, and K.

HOW TO DO IT:
- Avoid factory-made foods.
- Avoid foods wrapped in plastic.
- Avoid premade or ready-to-eat meals.

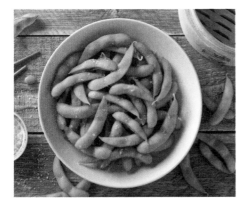

## PLANT-BASED PAIRINGS

Try these food combinations to provide your body with all necessary amino acids, fiber, and other nutrients you require to stay fit—especially if you aim to increase the ratio of plant-based dishes in your diet.

- Chopped red peppers and cooked cauliflower
- Carrots and lima beans
- Mustard greens and chickpeas
- Natural peanut butter and whole wheat bread
- Brown rice and edamame
- Extra-firm tofu and soba noodles

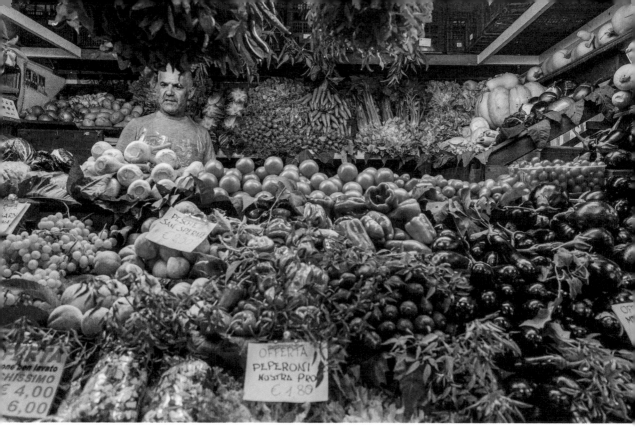

Fruits and vegetables are piled high at the San Benedetto market in the Sardinian city of Cagliari.

- Shop for foods at local farmers markets or community-supported farms.
- Try to eat at least three blue zones foods daily. These include beans of all kinds; greens such as spinach, kale, chard, beet tops, and fennel fronds; sweet potatoes; nuts; green extra-virgin olive oil; slow-cook or Irish steel-cut oats; barley in soups, as a hot cereal, or ground in bread; fruits; green and herbal teas; and turmeric as a spice or a tea.

## Drink mostly water

With very few exceptions, people in the blue zones drink coffee, tea, water, and wine. Period. Soft drinks are unknown to them. Tea is the drink enjoyed most among the longevity all-stars, whether it's black, green, or herbal.

Ikarians often brew tea from wild herbs, which may offer specific beneficial effects: Wild mint is used to prevent gingivitis and ulcers; rosemary to treat gout; artemisias to improve blood circulation. When I was in Ikaria, I sent samples of herbal tea to be laboratory-tested and found that they all had antioxidant properties in addition to functioning as mild diuretics. So they not only contain powerful antioxidants, but they also can help flush waste products from the body and slightly lower blood pressure.

Adventists, meanwhile, recommend drinking seven glasses of water daily. They point to studies that show that being hydrated facilitates blood flow and lessens the chance of a blood clot. Sardinians, Ikarians, and Nicoyans all drink copious amounts of coffee. Research links coffee drinking with lower rates of dementia and Parkinson's disease. People in most blue zones drink one to three small glasses of red wine per day, often with a meal and with friends.

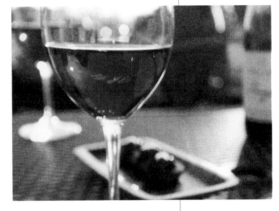

Most important, never drink soft drinks (including diet soda). Soft drinks account for about half of America's sugar intake. Instead, discover your favorite tea, be it rosemary, oregano, mint, sage, or some other herb. Then drink it daily.

People who drink red wine (in moderation) tend to outlive those who don't.

HOW TO DO IT:

- Keep a full water bottle at work and by your bed.
- Start the day with a cup of coffee. Avoid coffee after midafternoon, as caffeine can interfere with sleep.
- Sip green tea all day. It usually contains about 25 percent as much caffeine as coffee does.
- Try a variety of herbal teas, such as rosemary, oregano, or sage.
- Sweeten tea lightly with honey. Keep it in a pitcher in the fridge in hot weather.
- Never bring soft drinks into your house.

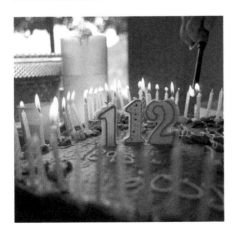

## CELEBRATE AND ENJOY FOOD

Eating the blue zones way may seem new to you. But it's not meant to feel like a restriction or limitation. Don't deprive yourself. Go ahead and enjoy the good meals and the occasional indulgent celebration.

- Pick one day of the week and make it your celebratory day to splurge on a meal with your favorite foods.
- Feel free to indulge at family celebrations and holidays. If it makes you feel happy, don't give up that slice of pie at Thanksgiving or that piece of birthday cake.

The trick is to painlessly find that happy balance between savoring our lives and behaving in a way that extends them.

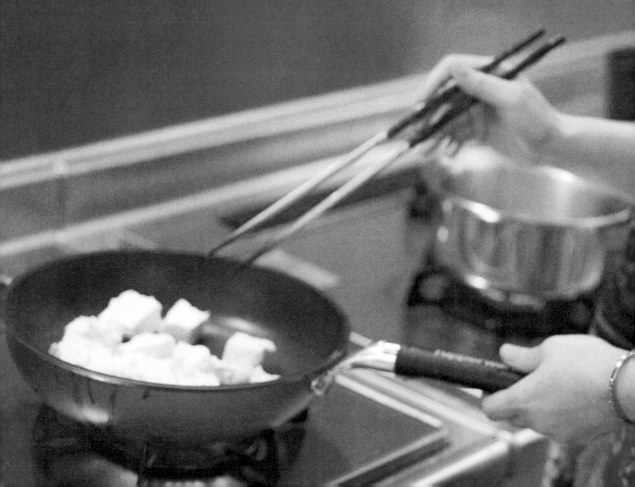

# CHAPTER 9

# Create Your
# Blue Zone

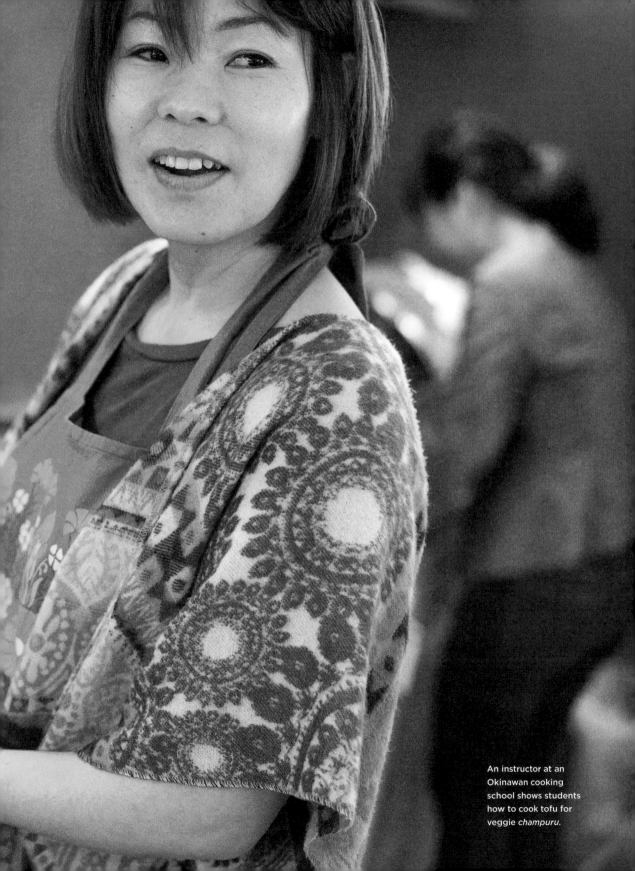

An instructor at an Okinawan cooking school shows students how to cook tofu for veggie *champuru*.

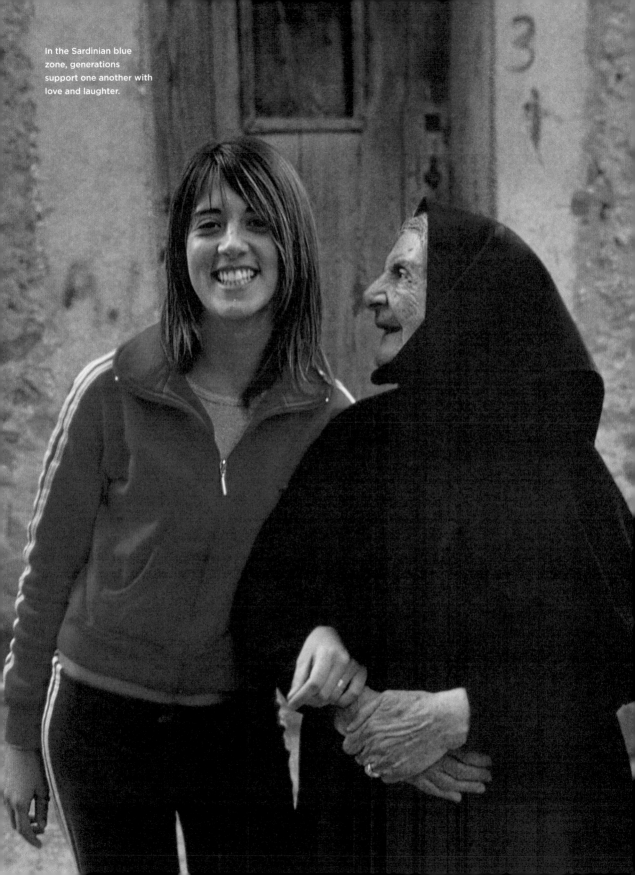

In the Sardinian blue zone, generations support one another with love and laughter.

# Design Your Surroundings

had an epiphany a few years ago. After visiting one of the world's blue zones, I realized that none of the spry centenarians I'd met there had *tried* to live into their 10th decade. Not one had taken stock of his or her life at middle age and said, "You know what, I'm going to get on a new diet, begin exercising, and maybe take a few supplements for a longer, healthier life."

Longevity just happened to them.

This idea was a game changer. I realized that the world's longest-lived people didn't follow a certain diet plan or possess outsized discipline, nor did they take greater responsibility for their health. Longevity happened to them almost naturally. It had flowed from their surroundings, a series of nudges and defaults that subtly and unconsciously helped them make the right choices—and avoid the wrong ones—for decades.

In the blue zones, streets are built for humans, not cars. Going to a friend's house, to work, to church, or out to eat is an opportunity for a walk. People still grind corn and knead bread by hand. They grow a garden.

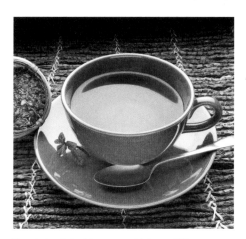

People in all the blue zones drink tea. Okinawans nurse green tea all day.

They aren't lonely, because it isn't an option. If after a few days people don't show up at the town festival, church, or even the village café, someone will generally check in on them. People talk face-to-face instead of by text, Facebook, or Snapchat. Blue zones residents have a sense of purpose, as well. Their lives are imbued with meaning from age 10 to age 100, and their brand of purpose isn't just hobbies or golf. It also includes a sense of responsibility for their community, their family, and the next generation.

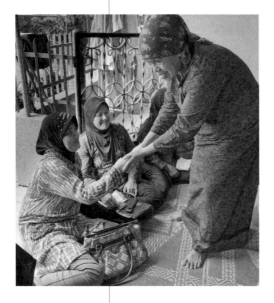

Members of an Indonesian family greet one another at a Sunday afternoon gathering.

Here in the United States, many of us have come to feel that there's something wrong with our way of life, the foods we consume, the frantic pace we keep, the relationships we make, and the communities we create—something that keeps us from being as happy and healthy as we could be. Our homes, neighborhoods, schools, workplaces, streets, and towns are set up to support convenience—including fast, calorie-rich, and nutrient-poor foods and a life spent sitting (at your desk, in your car, on your couch)—rather than well-being. To create our personal blue zones, we must reengineer our surroundings to replicate the time-honored practices we know support health and longevity.

In the blue zones, people move naturally all day, have strong social support systems, and eat healthy foods most of the time because their environments nudge them to do so all day, every day. Scientists at the Mayo Clinic have estimated that increasing simple movements such as standing and walking can help you burn an additional 350 calories a day. By optimizing your home, they say you can burn an extra 150 calories a day, which could add up to six fewer pounds in a year.

To bring these benefits to Americans, we've launched community makeover projects in more than 72 cities and states across the country in what's been

## LIFE RADIUS

The blue zone approach to making our communities stronger and healthier focuses on our "life radius," the area close to home where we spend 90 percent of our lives.

- **The built environment:** Improve roads and transportation options, parks, and public spaces.
- **Municipal policies and ordinances:** Promote activity and discourage junk-food marketing and smoking.

- **Restaurants, schools, grocery stores, faith-based organizations, and workplaces:** Build healthy options into the places people spend the most time.
- **Social networks:** Form and nurture social groups that support healthy habits.
- **Habitat:** Help people design homes that nudge them into eating less and moving more.
- **Inner selves:** Encourage people to reduce stress, find their purpose, and give back to the community.

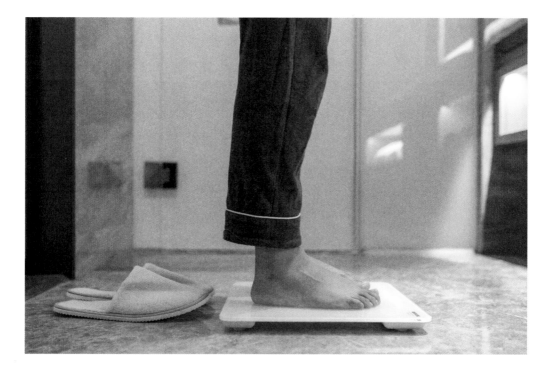

described as "the biggest healthy living experiment" in the nation. We're helping to tweak whole towns so that people don't have to think about being healthier, because their communities are built to get them there. We want people to love what they eat, how they spend their days, and the people they spend time with. We want them to feel that their lives are getting better, whether they start by embracing blue zones ideas on a small scale at home or become inspired to transform their entire neighborhood, town, or city.

In this chapter, we'll show you how to set up your own surroundings with nudges and defaults so that the healthy choice is always the easy choice.

People who step on a scale daily tend to weigh less than those who don't.

## Setting Up Your Home

Many simple decisions you make about the design of your house and the pathway of your everyday life affect your health and longevity. If you live in a home that is full of nudges that keep you moving, you're not only burning more calories with physical activity; you're also keeping your metabolism working at a higher rate. This natural movement creates a heart-healthy, fat-burning blood chemistry that keeps you sharper and feeling more energetic. From the kitchen to your bedroom, into the yard, and out into your community, here are some changes you can make right now to create your own blue zone.

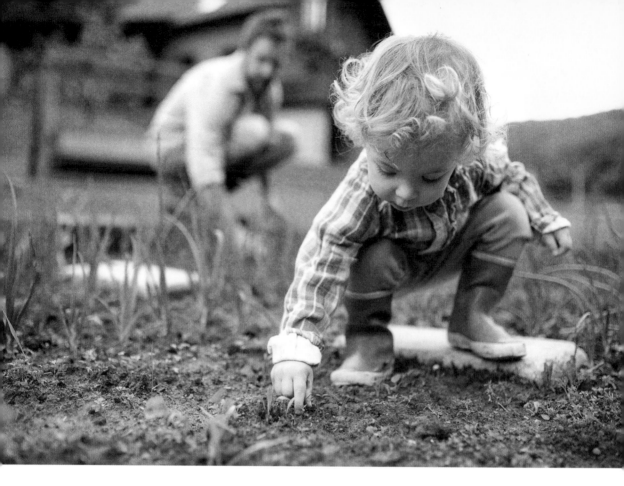

A young gardener and her father thin out seedlings and pluck weeds in the family plot.

- **Place your scale in a visible place and use it daily.** If you don't have a scale, buy an inexpensive one. It doesn't need all the bells and whistles. People who weigh themselves every day for two years weigh as much as 17 pounds less after two years than people who never weigh themselves. Daily weight checks take only seconds, and the results can provide powerful reinforcement.

- **Have only one TV in your home.** Put it in a common room, preferably in a cabinet behind doors. The goal here is to nudge you away from screen time that encourages overeating and detracts from potential physical activity. People who watch too much TV are more likely to be overweight. Watching TV actually lowers metabolism, makes us less active and engaged, and encourages us to eat junk food via commercials. Kids with a TV in their bedrooms are 18 percent more likely to be (or become) obese and have lower grades. The happiest people watch only 30 to 60 minutes of TV per day.

- **Replace power tools with hand tools.** Shoveling, raking, and pushing a mower are healthy and productive outdoor workouts—some burn almost 400 calories an hour. In fact, mowing the lawn or raking leaves burns about the same number of calories as lifting weights. If you are able, mow your lawn with a push lawn mower, shovel the snow with a hand shovel, and gather the leaves from your lawn with an old-fashioned rake instead of a leaf blower.

■ **Grow and maintain your own garden or plants.** In all blue zones, people continue to garden even into their 90s and 100s. Gardening is the epitome of a blue zones activity because it's sort of a nudge: You plant the seeds and you're going to be nudged in the next three to four months to water the plants, weed them, harvest them. Gardening also provides low-intensity range-of-motion exercise, vitamin D from the sun, and fresh vegetables and herbs. Watering plants burns about the same number of calories as stretching and walking. Studies show that working with plants can also reduce psychological and physiological stress.

We recommend that you plant a garden in your yard, start a container garden on your patio, cultivate an indoor herb garden on your windowsill, or add indoor plants into your home. For indoor plants that are easy to maintain, try a golden pothos vine or a spider plant. Besides their ability to clean the air, indoor plants have been proved to provide health benefits to people who interact with them. And because plants are permanent, you'll be nudged to nurture them daily.

■ **Welcome a dog into your family.** If you and your family are prepared to care for a dog, consider adopting or buying one. Pets make great companions and encourage you to walk or run. Researchers found that if you own a dog, you naturally get over five hours of exercise a week. In fact, studies have shown that dog owners have lower rates of health problems, compared with those

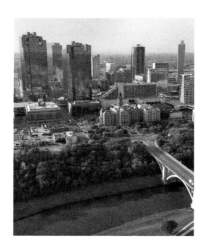

### COWTOWN MAKES A COMEBACK

In 2014 the city of Fort Worth, Texas, ranked near the bottom of the Gallup-Sharecare Index of overall well-being—185th out of 190 communities in the United States. Four years later, after embracing a Blue Zones Project, the city jumped to 58th. How did the city do it? By making changes to its environment—its workplaces, schools, restaurants, grocery stores, parks, and streets—that nudged residents into healthy behaviors. As a result, 31 percent fewer people in Fort Worth are smoking, and 62 percent more are staying active on 87 miles of new bike lanes and trails, sidewalks, gardens, and workplaces. Children have joined running clubs in schools, restaurants have adopted healthier items on their menus, and supermarkets have created blue zone checkout lanes with nutritious items.

who don't own a dog. (Although you don't walk them, there are some research-backed health benefits to owning a cat and other types of pets as well.)

■ Own a bike. Buy a bike or fix your current bike so you can use it. Just having a bike nudges you to use it. Riding at a moderate speed burns approximately 235 calories per half hour. Be sure to buy a good helmet. Wearing a bicycle helmet reduces the risk of serious head injury in crashes by as much as 85 percent, and the risk for brain injury by as much as 88 percent.

■ Own at least four of the following: walking shoes, jump rope, yoga mat, weights, basketball, football, golf clubs, Rollerblades, camping supplies, running shoes. Having walking and exercise equipment in your home encourages physical activity. Make sure this equipment is easy to use. Roller-blading burns more calories than running track and field hurdles, and playing catch for only 30 minutes burns over 100 calories.

■ Create an indoor exercise area. Exercising is more convenient when you have a space in your home designated for that purpose. You are more likely to use the equipment if it's easily accessible and visible. A study at the University of Florida found that women who exercised at home lost 25 pounds in 15 months and maintained that loss. Designate a portion or a corner of a room in your home for your exercise equipment, stability ball, yoga mat, and/or weight set.

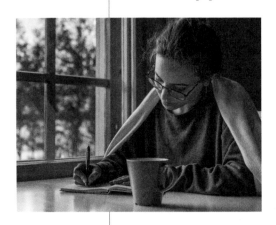

Keeping a journal can boost your happiness, relieve stress, and improve your memory.

■ Place cushions on the floor. Instead of sitting on chairs and furniture all the time, create an area where you can sit on cushions on the floor for reading, talking on the phone, relaxing, enjoying hobbies, or doing family activities. Okinawan elders sit and get up from the floor dozens of times per day. This exercises their legs, back, and core in a routine way. Sitting on the floor also improves posture and increases overall strength, flexibility, and mobility. Supporting yourself without a chairback improves posture and may help you burn up to an additional 130 calories each hour.

■ Create a family "pride shrine" area or wall. A "pride shrine" is a place with family photos, mementos, and objects that display your accomplishments. Put it in a high-traffic area in your home, maybe between your bedroom and your bathroom, and every time you walk by, you'll be rewarded with a surge

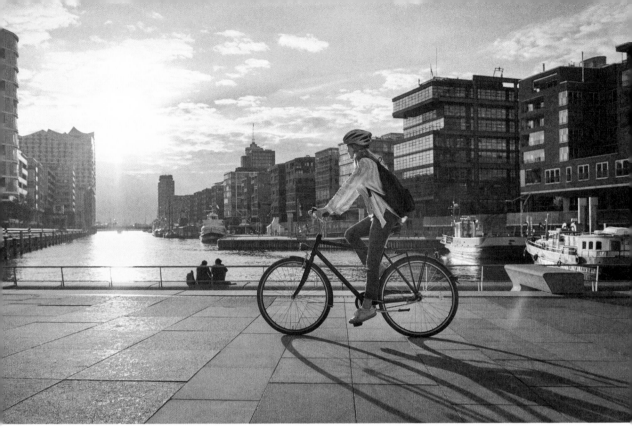

of pride and a reminder of how you fit into the world. It can be pictures of your kids when they were young, a remembrance of a parent or a grandparent, pictures of your vacation spot, diplomas, and articles that you've liked.

- **Create a destination room.** Include a large table for family projects, shelves filled with books, and plenty of light. Keep out the clock, TV, computer, or other distracting gadgets.
- **Disconnect your garage door opener.** Instead, get out of the car and open the door manually.

## Setting Up Your Kitchen

For most of their lives, the world's longest-lived peoples ate whole, plant-based foods, and their kitchens were set up to make those foods taste good. They stocked their kitchens with hand-operated equipment that made preparing and cooking food a more physical and meditative process.

To create your own blue zones kitchen, there are four simple things you can do. First, keep the healthiest ingredients on hand and in plain sight. Second, equip your kitchen with cookware and utensils that enable you to make delicious, healthy foods quickly. Third, make safety your top priority. And

Biking is a great way to keep active and reduce stress.

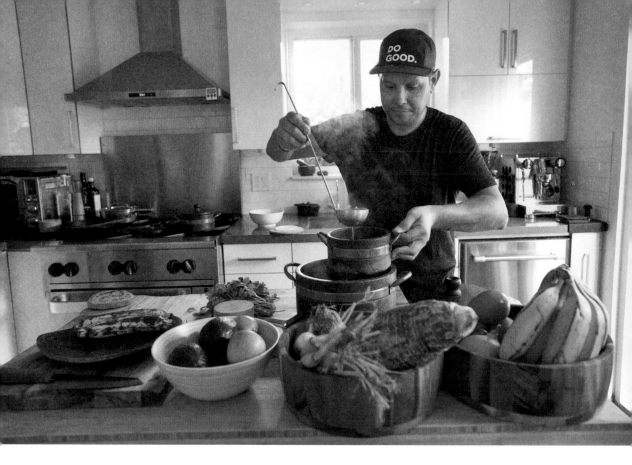

Diego Tosoni, a Miami-based chef, practices vegan cooking at home and at his restaurant, Love Life Cafe.

fourth, develop the habit of using nonmechanized appliances to keep you moving naturally while you cook.

- **Optimize your layout.** The most efficient kitchens are set up with the stove, sink, and refrigerator as points of a triangle. Ideally, the sink sits next to the stove on one side and the refrigerator on the other. This layout optimizes efficiency and will help make cooking more enjoyable. Think about your own workflow and access patterns, positioning movable things such as cutting boards and placing equipment like pots, pans, and flatware where they are most convenient.

- **Invest in the right refrigerator.** A new, smaller refrigerator may be a good health investment. Why new? Because the latest models keep fruit, vegetables, and other food fresher longer by eliminating bacteria and gases more efficiently, thus hindering spoilage. Why smaller? Studies have shown that the more food you have in your refrigerator, the more you're likely to eat. A small refrigerator can serve as a nudge to eat less—and encourage you to go shopping for fresh food more often.

- **Clear plenty of counter space.** You will feel best about cooking if you have a large, inviting space on which to chop and prepare your food. (Put your TV and mail somewhere else.)
- **Get good lighting.** To enjoy preparing food, make sure your prep space has plenty of light. Eyestrain can be a negative nudge, subconsciously driving you away from cooking. Consider adding under-the-cabinet lighting in darker kitchens to brighten your space even more.
- **Keep a small pantry.** Our grandparents used to store homemade conserves, pickled vegetables, and fruit jams in their pantries. Today's pantries are more likely to carry gigantic bags of chips and pretzels, cases of granola bars, and boxes of cereals. One study found that people who cooked using ingredients from large containers prepared 23 percent more food—a good reason to leave the 25-pound bag of rice at the warehouse club.

## Kitchen Checklist

Begin by decluttering your pantry, kitchen, and refrigerator, and clearing your countertops of snack foods (that open bag of chips, that box of crackers). Physically remove foods that are off-limits or too tempting, such as candy and junk or processed items. Create an inconvenient junk-food cabinet or drawer

### KITCHEN EQUIPMENT CHECKLIST

Having the right tools can make all the difference for busy cooks.

**Solid cutting board** Get the largest bamboo or wood board you have room for.

**Knives** Every kitchen should have an eight-inch chef's knife, a paring knife, and a serrated knife. Keep them sharpened.

**Mandoline slicer** Use it to slice vegetables like zucchini and potatoes.

**Wooden spoons** These bacteria-resistant implements make cooking easy.

**Cast-iron pans** Naturally nonstick once seasoned, they'll last a lifetime.

**Food mill** Use it to crush cooked vegetables and fruit for soup and sauces.

**Potato masher** It makes creamy mashed potatoes, a quick salsa, or a spread with cooked or canned beans.

**Box grater** Use it to shred fruits and vegetables. Hold it with one hand.

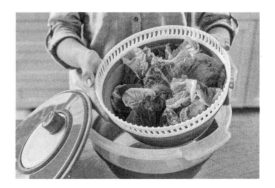

**Salad spinner** Dry lettuce and other leafy greens after washing.

**Food processor** It can chop veggies in a flash or make smooth dough or batter.

**Immersion blender** Puree soups right in the pot.

**Sieve or colander** Keep it within easy reach of the sink to rinse fruits and vegetables.

**Slow cooker** It can save you time and money. Turn it on low and forget about it.

that is up high or down low. Research shows that if it's out of sight and inconvenient, we'll eat less of it. Put your toaster away, too. A toaster on the counter provides a visual clue to toast something every time you walk into the kitchen, and most of what we put into toasters is unhealthy.

Consider the following tips and see how many things you're already doing—and how many others you could do—to move yourself and your family toward greater health and longevity.

- **Keep fruits and vegetables at eye level in your refrigerator.** Dedicate the center section of your refrigerator to healthy foods that encourage you to snack mindfully.
- **Keep unhealthy snacks out of sight—on a top or bottom shelf or inside a drawer or cabinet you don't often open.** Label the shelf or drawer "Junk Food." Most junk food is consumed because you see it and it looks good. If you're going to have junk food in your house, hide it from your line of vision to decrease consumption.
- **Put a fresh fruit bowl on the kitchen table or in another prominent spot.** The first thing you see when you walk through your kitchen should be something healthy. Never put chips or packaged sweets in plain view.
- **Use dinner plates no larger than 10 inches across.** Put away your larger plates. Eating on smaller plates creates the perception of more generous portions and tricks the brain into being satisfied with less food.
- **Drink beverages out of tall, narrow glasses—no more than 2.5 inches in diameter.** We visually measure our drinks by height, not width, of the glass. Narrow glasses make us think we are drinking more than we actually are.
- **Plate your entire meal and put leftovers away before sitting down at the table.** Consider putting a "Dish Here, Dine There" reminder note on the counter next to the stove. People who prepare food consume less.
- **Remove the TV, cell phones, and computers from the kitchen and dining rooms.** Create a no-electronics zone. Watching TV, listening to fast-paced music, and using electronic devices all promote mindless eating. TVs also take up important countertop space in your kitchen.

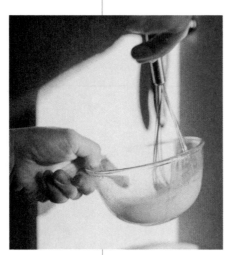

Using hand-operated kitchen tools keeps you moving naturally while you cook.

- **Use hand-operated kitchen tools.** Get rid of your electric can opener and use a hand-operated one instead. Get a potato masher, a garlic press, and whisk, rather than using a blender or electric mixer. Try squeezing fruit juice by hand.
- **Buy an electric pressure cooker.** A generic type is fine, or you could try a name brand like Instant Pot. Buy microwave-safe food storage containers (I like Pyrex) or recycle glass pasta sauce jars, pickle jars, or other glass bottles for leftovers and meal prep.
- **Hang up the "Four Always, Four to Avoid" list in your kitchen.** The "Always" foods are the ones you want to keep on hand. They should be readily available, affordable, taste good, and be versatile enough to include in most meals. The "Avoid" foods are those that have been highly correlated with obesity, heart disease, or cancer, as well as causing constant temptations in the average American diet.

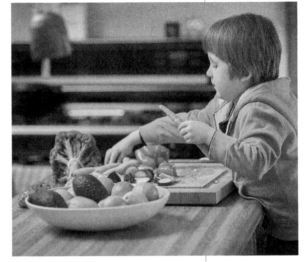

Place a bowl of fresh fruits and veggies in a prominent place for snacking.

## Four Always

### 1. 100 percent whole grains

These include oats, barley, brown rice, and corn, as well as farro, quinoa, whole cornmeal, and bulgur wheat. About 65 percent of the diets in the blue zones consist of whole grains, beans, and starchy tubers. Meta-analysis reviews (studies of studies) found that consuming whole grains reduces your risk of diseases that shorten your life.

### 2. Nuts

Eat two handfuls per day. A handful of nuts weighs about two ounces, the average amount that blue zones centenarians consume. Keep a can of your favorite nuts in your office or house as your most convenient snack.

### 3. Beans

Beans and legumes are the cornerstone of every longevity diet in the world. We recommend that you eat a cup of cooked beans per day.

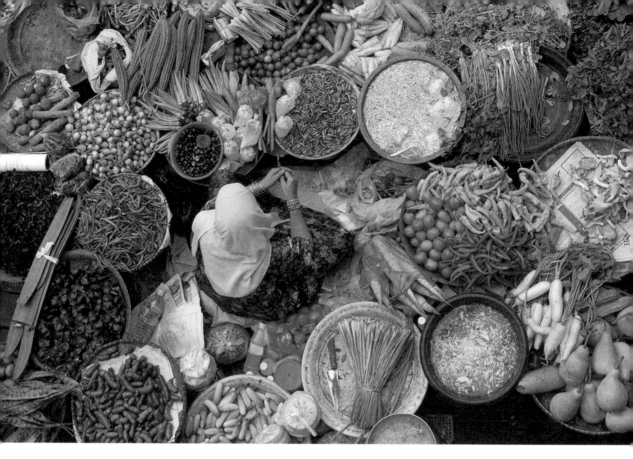

A market stall in Kota Bharu, Malaysia, displays a wide variety of fresh vegetables.

### 4. Your favorite fruits and vegetables

Research suggests that people who eat five fruits and vegetables a day live an extra three years, compared with their non-plant-eating counterparts. Eating seven or more portions of fruit and vegetables a day can lower your risk of premature death by a whopping 42 percent. And even though some fruits and vegetables are healthier than others (berries are better than bananas), we suggest you stock up on your favorites because you're more likely to actually eat them.

## Four to Avoid

### 1. Sugar-sweetened beverages

These empty calories are the number one source of refined sugars in the American diet.

### 2. Salty snacks

Salty snacks are not only high in sodium, but they're also fattening. Salty snacks are one of the foods most associated with obesity.

### 3. Packaged sweets

Cookies, candies, and processed sweets are also highly associated with obesity. Sugar is arguably the number one toxin in the American diet.

### 4. Processed meats

The World Health Organization puts processed meats in the same category as cigarette smoking—a known carcinogen.

Remove "Avoid" foods from your house: Throw out the soda and other sugar-sweetened beverages, candy, chips, cookies, bacon, and sausages. Stock up on "Always" foods like beans, nuts, grains, fruits, and vegetables. We prefer dried beans and fresh vegetables, but low-sodium canned versions are also OK. Although less-processed whole grains like brown rice, barley, and quinoa are better, 100 percent whole-grain products like whole wheat bread and whole wheat pasta are OK, too. Do some meal planning for the week so that grocery shopping is easy.

## Setting Up Your Bedroom

The keys to enjoying a restful night are establishing a relaxing bedroom routine and creating a bedroom environment that provides a sanctuary for sleep. In the blue zones, most centenarians go to bed shortly after sunset and wake with daybreak, which gives them eight hours of sleep. In at least three of the blue zones, a half-hour nap is also a daily ritual—very different from our routines.

Americans today report an average of 6.8 hours of sleep a day, according to Gallup. Fourteen percent sleep fewer than six hours. That's not enough. As research shows, lack of sleep increases one's risk of health problems,

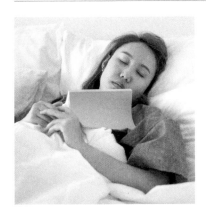

### HEALTH BENEFITS OF SLEEP

When you get enough restful sleep, you think better, process information more easily, and have a more positive outlook. By contrast, chronic sleep disruption makes you more prone to depression. During sleep, your blood pressure decreases, giving your heart and blood vessels time to rest and repair. Deep sleep also induces a drop in blood sugar levels. With better blood sugar regulation, you're less likely to develop type 2 diabetes. Getting enough sleep also supports your immune system and helps regulate hormones that control appetite. When sleep is disrupted, you may be more prone to overeat or to eat junk food.

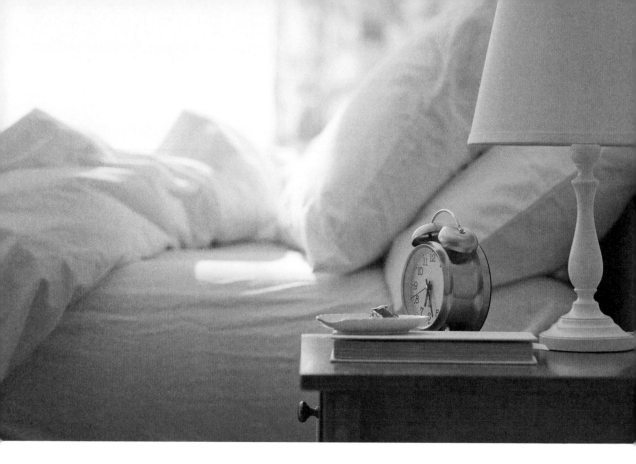

**Set up a regular bedtime routine, eat well, and get enough exercise to prevent sleep problems.**

including obesity, diabetes, cardiovascular disease, and hypertension. It can also lead to impaired judgment, risky decision making, and even decreased attractiveness.

Blue Zones bedrooms are cool, quiet, and dark. There are no computers, TVs, or cell phones. People don't use alarm clocks. No one is jolted awake at 2 a.m. by text messages or incoming emails. Because they sleep enough, they wake up naturally.

## Bedroom Checklist

The following suggestions were developed in collaboration with the Cornell Center for Sleep Medicine. Its doctors take their cues from the blue zones and couple them with evidence-based information on how to improve your bedroom and sleeping habits.

■ **Own a comfortable mattress and pillows.** Make sure that your mattress doesn't sag and that it supports you comfortably as you sleep. Replace your mattress every eight to 10 years. When choosing a mattress, spend at least 10 minutes lying on it to test it out before buying it. Choose comfortable pillows that support your head without crimping your neck.

- **Make your bedroom cool at night.** Set your thermostat to 65°F at bedtime. If you have a programmable thermostat, have it automatically adjust to that temperature during sleeping hours. Temperatures below 54°F or about 75°F can actually wake you up at night. If 65°F feels a little cooler than you'd like, add a blanket.

- **Dim the lights an hour before bedtime.** Try to get into the habit of dimming all the lights in your home an hour before you go to bed. It prepares your body for sleep and allows you to fall asleep faster and stay asleep longer. It's also a step toward the darkness you need (which is explained in the next item).

- **Remove digital alarm clocks with lit-up screens.** Even the LED lights from clocks can suppress melatonin, a hormone that helps promote sleep. Hiding your clock from your line of sight will also help you avoid obsessive clock watching during the night.

- **Use shades, blinds, or drapery to block outside light.** Light, including city streetlights or outdoor security lights, can disrupt sleep. Hang light-blocking window shades or heavy drapery that can block out all outside light to make your room as dark as possible for the best sleep.

- **Remove the TV, computer, and cell phones from the bedroom.** Treat your bedroom as a no-electronics zone. By removing the light sources and distractions, you are creating an environment conducive to calmness and a deeper, more restful, and healthful sleep.

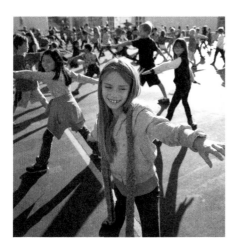

### KEEPING FIT IN THE BEACH CITIES

Three communities in Southern California—Hermosa Beach, Redondo Beach, and Manhattan Beach—are doing something about childhood obesity, a problem that afflicts one in five American youths. As part of a Blue Zones Project demonstration, these cities recommitted to promoting healthier environments for their kids by nudging them into physical activity and better eating and also by providing healthier school meals, morning exercise activities, classroom activity breaks, a walking school-bus program, a program for preschoolers, bicycle safety education, and mindfulness activities. The results: From 2009 to 2017, obesity among schoolchildren in Redondo Beach fell from 13.9 percent to 6.4 percent.

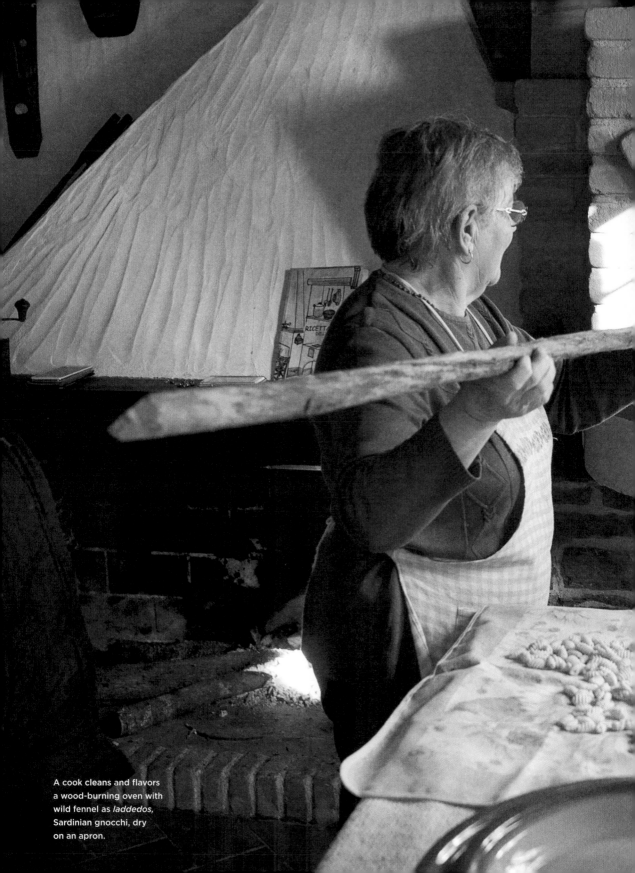

A cook cleans and flavors a wood-burning oven with wild fennel as *laddedos,* Sardinian gnocchi, dry on an apron.

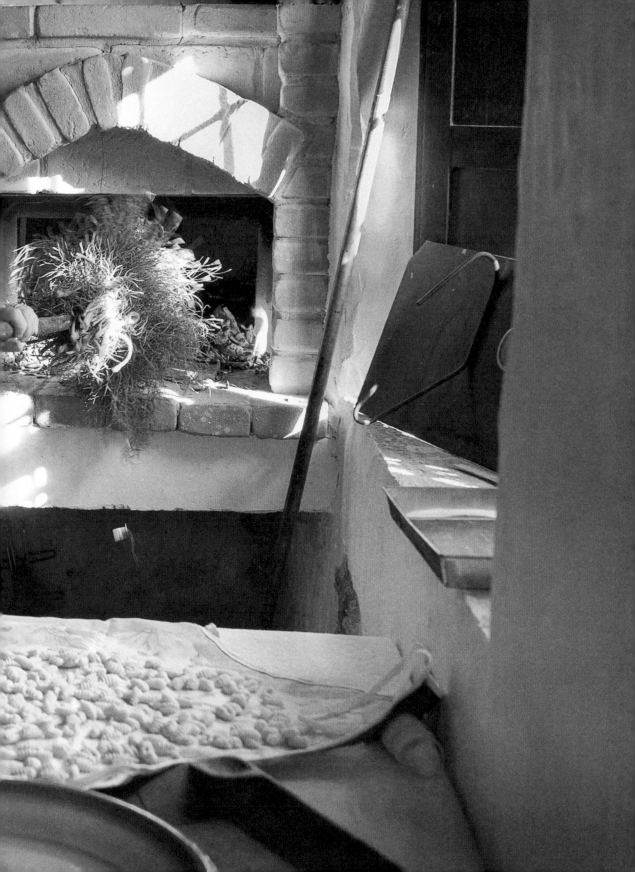

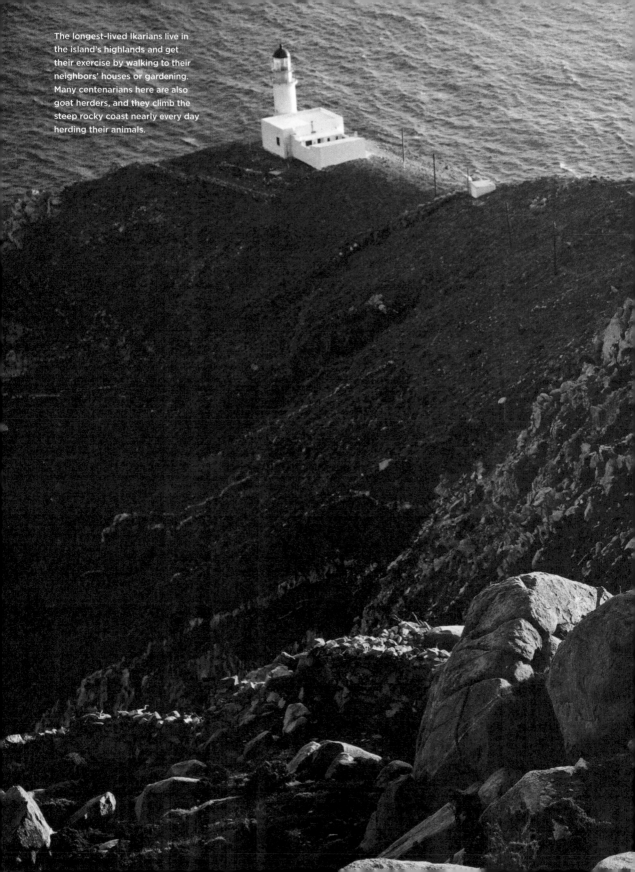

The longest-lived Ikarians live in the island's highlands and get their exercise by walking to their neighbors' houses or gardening. Many centenarians here are also goat herders, and they climb the steep rocky coast nearly every day herding their animals.

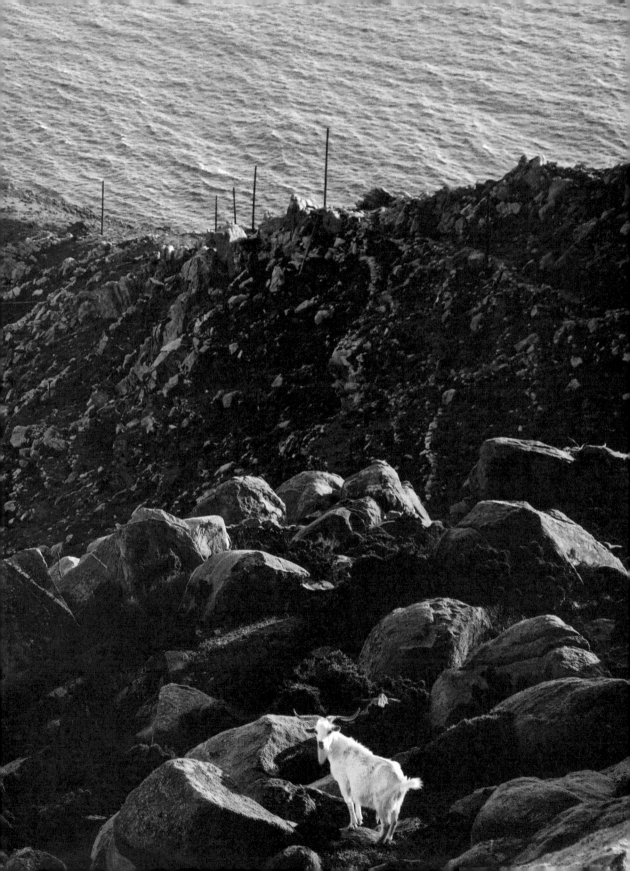

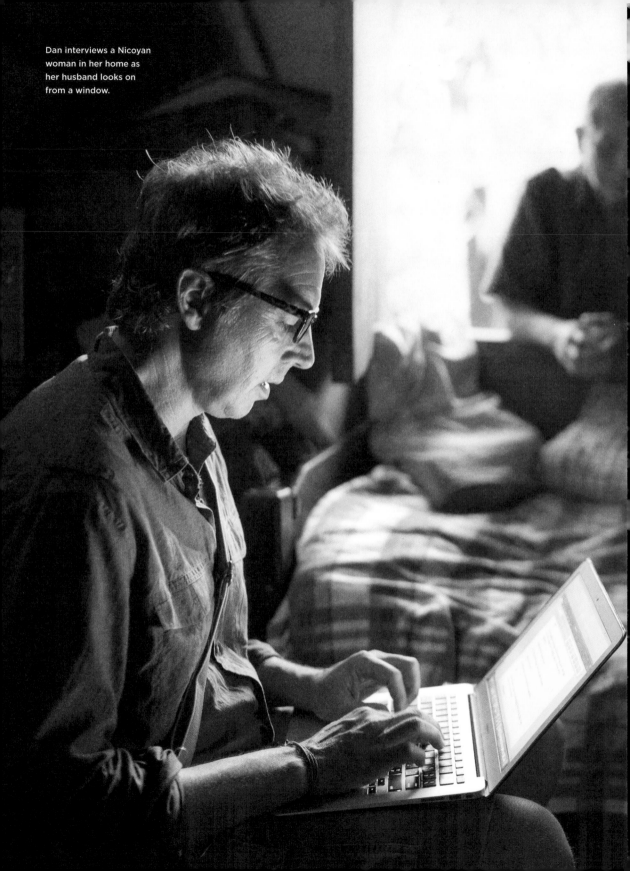

Dan interviews a Nicoyan woman in her home as her husband looks on from a window.

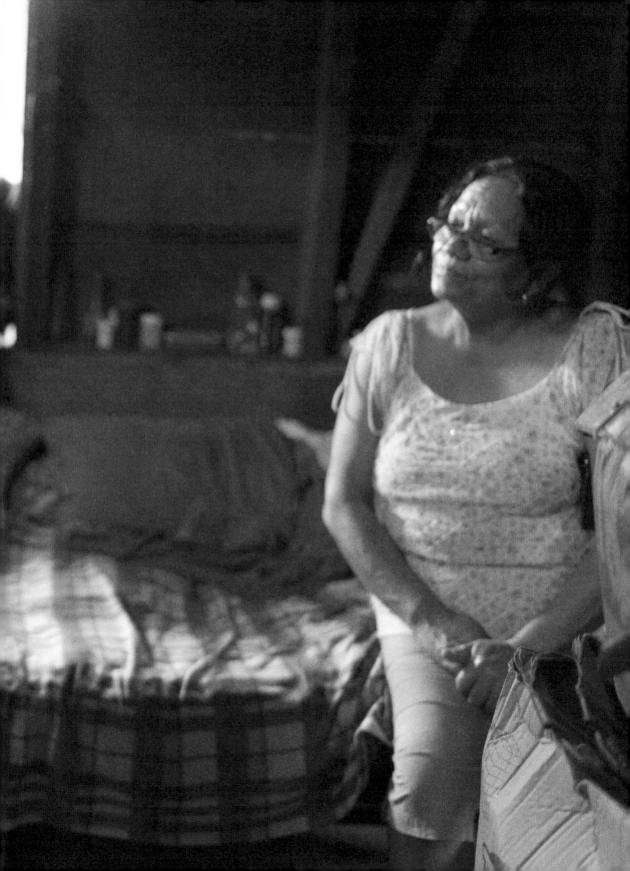

# Living Long and Well

A few years ago, while on assignment for *National Geographic,* I met one of the happiest men on Earth. Statistically speaking, I knew the profile called for a healthy, middle-age father living in a place like Costa Rica with engaging work. After much searching, I narrowed it down to a 57-year-old roving avocado salesman named Alejandro Zuñiga.

I met Alejandro at the central market in the city of Cartago. A sprawling boisterous bazaar, the market buzzed with tropical produce vendors who endlessly heckled customers—and each other—for business.

Alejandro moved through the stalls like a charismatic tarpon in a school of sardines, shaking hands, asking after family, and exchanging jokes. He was a natural leader, and people loved him. He organized bus trips for soccer games and fundraisers for vendors down on their luck. But when it came to business, he was a disaster and perpetually broke.

A few years earlier, at the end of a long day of pushing his avocado cart around with little luck, he heard his flip phone ring. "You won the lottery!" shouted one of his market pals. "The big one!" Alejandro was down to his last eight dollars and not amused at what he took to be a joke.

He hung up. His friend promptly called back and confirmed the news.

Alejandro had won 50 million colones (about $82,000 today)—enough money to live out the rest of his life comfortably. But he didn't do that. A few weeks later, he was back in the market with his avocados. He began giving away his money—to the soup vendor who used to comp him lunch, to a lady who lost her husband, to friends who asked for loans, to his mother. When I met him, he was broke again. Yet he insisted, "I couldn't be happier."

Why am I telling this story? Because there's an ever growing industry (estimated to be worth $182 billion by 2028) selling us the promise of "antiaging" and longevity. But it misses the point of living.

Sure, there are lots of promising treatments. Testosterone therapy is said to restore vigor and build muscle in older men. Metformin—a drug commonly used to treat people with diabetes—seems to restore metabolic vitality for couch potatoes (although it offers no additional benefit for people who exercise).

In his excellent book *The Great Age Reboot,* Dr. Michael Roizen outlines 14 scientific advancements that could extend our lives by decades, or even "make 90 the new 40." These include

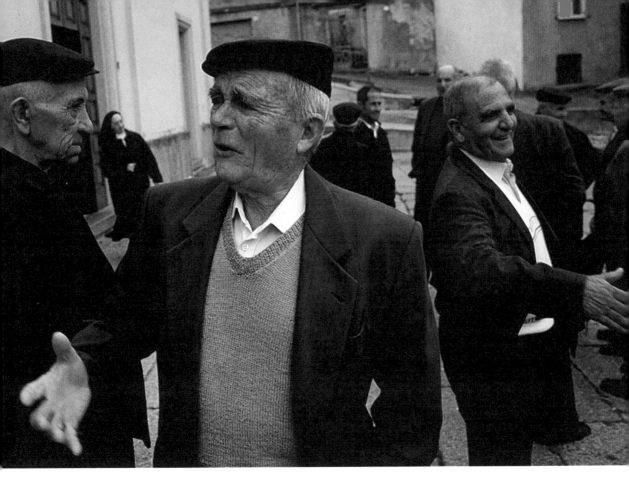

Sardinian men greet one another in a mountain village. Studies show that socializing promotes both longevity and happiness.

injecting our bodies with young cells that can reprogram old cells and genetic splicing that can instruct our genes to rejuvenate tissue. Are any of them a sure shot? No. But he puts the chance at 80 percent that at least one of them will work in extending our lives.

Still, the first interventions are more likely to slow aging than to reverse it. And none of them promises to help us enjoy the journey.

Most of what fuels a long life in the blue zones also happens to produce a good life. The people who live there are not only the statistically longest lived but also among the happiest on Earth. Besides being home to the Nicoya blue zone, for example, Costa Rica produces the world's happiest lives per GDP dollar.

As Alejandro illustrates, people who possess generosity, a strong sense of purpose, a rich social life, and move naturally all day long enjoy a manifest boost in happiness. These are the same factors that have helped people in the world's blue zones live record-breaking long lives.

So, while there's a fair chance that in your lifetime some scientific breakthrough may come along to extend your life, your best bet for longevity and happiness is still to follow the lessons from the blue zones. And now you have a how-to manual.

*To Brooke and Maverick Buettner, born into a generation—and a family—*
*who may be the first to routinely reach 100.*

This book required another shockingly enormous effort by a multidisciplinary team, many of whom put in just as much time and effort as I did.

My longtime *National Geographic* editor, Peter Miller, did the vast majority of shaping my notes into this book. If it's a success, he gets much of the credit. Almost two decades ago, I came to *National Geographic* with an idea to reverse engineer longevity by finding longevity hot spots. If Peter had not taken a flier and assigned me the story, the Blue Zones phenomenon might have never happened. Thank you, Pedro!

This book grew out of my experiences while shooting a Blue Zones series for Netflix in collaboration with MakeMake Entertainment. I have to thank Angus Wall and Kent Kubena for guiding the vision and selling it to Netflix. Director Clay Jeter and producer Rich Eckersley are the smartest, most uncharacteristically generous collaborators I could imagine. They are master storytellers. Also, thanks to brilliant researcher Chamberlain Staub, who always found the proverbial needle in the academic haystack. And a special thanks to producer Amanda Rohlke, the hardest-working and most productive human I've ever encountered, who literally worked around the clock during the four-month shoot.

My longtime photographic partner, David McLain, brought this book to life visually. David has been with me every step of this Blue Zones journey, helping me think through every facet of the stories. He, in fact, suggested I name the project Blue Zones. Thank you, Big Shooter!

My chief of staff, Sam Skemp, managed the storm of details, from travel to research coordination. Thank you for your relentless loyalty, unflappability, and hard work.

At National Geographic, Adrian Coakley, Jill Foley, and Molly Roberts worked with David to wade through more than 20,000 frames to choose the images for this book. I'd also like to thank senior editor Allyson Johnson, creative director Elisa Gibson, senior production editor Michael O'Connor, director of communications Ann Day, and especially editorial director and publisher Lisa Thomas, who originally saw the potential of a book titled *Blue Zones*.

At the Blue Zones office, I'm grateful for the help of April Lunde, Aislinn Kotifani, Nick Buettner, Amelia Clabots, Danny Buettner-Salido, and especially CEO Ben Leedle for their support and logistical help.

Few get far in life without support from close friends. I want to thank Kevin Moore, Remar Sutton, Jon Norberg, Gayle Winegar, John Mackey, Matthew McConaughey, Matthew O'Hayer, Alexander Green, Mark and Penelope Greene, Pilar Gerasimo, Tom Boesen, Varda Nauen, Rudy Maxa, Rob Perez, Ellie Andersen, and Stephanie Blanda for supporting me during the writing of this book. And I am especially grateful for my parents, Roger and Dolly Buettner, who continue to support me to this day.

## INTRODUCTION

Herskind, A. M., et al. "The Heritability of Human Longevity: A Population-Based Study of 2,872 Danish Twin Pairs Born 1870–1900." In *Human Genetics* 97 (March 1996).

Hjelmborg, J., et al. "Genetic Influence on Human Lifespan and Longevity." In *Human Genetics* 119, no. 3 (April 2006).

Olshansky, S. Jay, et al. "Position Statement on Human Aging." In *Journals of Gerontology Series A: Biological Sciences and Medical Sciences* 57, no. 8 (August 2002).

## CHAPTER 1: SARDINIA

Deiana, L., et al. "AKEntAnnos: The Sardinia Study of Extreme Longevity." In *Aging* 11, no. 3 (June 1999).

Hitchcott, P. K., et al. "Psychological Well-Being in Italian Families: An Exploratory Approach to the Study of Mental Health Across the Adult Life Span in the Blue Zone." In *European Journal of Psychology* 13, no. 3 (August 2017).

Pes, G., F. Tolu, M. P. Dore, et al. "Male Longevity in Sardinia, a Review of Historical Sources Supporting a Causal Link with Dietary Factors." In *European Journal of Clinical Nutrition* 69, no. 4 (April 2015).

Pes, G., F. Tolu, M. Poulain, et al. "Lifestyle and Nutrition Related to Male Longevity in Sardinia: An Ecological Study." In *Nutrition, Metabolism, and Cardiovascular Diseases* 23, no. 3 (March 2013).

Poulain, M., G. Pes, and L. Salaris. "A Population Where Men Live as Long as Women: Villagrande Strisaili, Sardinia." In *Journal of Aging Research* 2011 (June 2011).

Poulain, M., G. M. Pes, C. Grasland, et al. "Identification of a Geographic Area Characterized by Extreme Longevity in the Sardinia Island: The AKEA study." In *Experimental Gerontology* 39, no. 9 (September 2004).

## CHAPTER 2: NICOYA

Flores, M. "Food Patterns in Central America and Panama." In *Tradition, Science, and Practice in Dietetics: Proceedings of the 3rd International Congress of Dietetics,* London, July 10–14. Newman Books, 1961.

Gawande, Atul. "Costa Ricans Live Longer Than We Do. What's the Secret?" In *The New Yorker,* August 23, 2021.

Rehkopf, D. H., et al. "Longer Leukocyte Telomere Length in Costa Rica's Nicoya Peninsula: A Population-Based Study." In *Experimental Gerontology* 48, no. 11 (November 2013).

Rosero-Bixby, L. "Assessing the Impact of Health Sector Reform in Costa Rica Through a Quasi-Experimental Study." In *Pan American Journal of Public Health* 15, no. 2 (February 2004).

———. "The Exceptionally High Life Expectancy of Costa Rican Nonagenarians." In *Demography* 45, no. 3 (August 2008).

Rosero-Bixby, L., and William H. Dow. "Exploring Why Costa Rica Outperforms the United States in Life Expectancy: A Tale of Two Inequality Gradients." In *PNAS* 113, no. 5 (February 2016).

Ruiz Narváez, E., et al. "Diet and Leukocyte Telomere Length in a Population With Extended Longevity: The Costa Rican Longevity and Healthy Aging Study (CRELES)." In *Nutrients* 13, no. 8 (July 2021).

## CHAPTER 3: LOMA LINDA

Fraser, G. E. "A Comparison of First Event Coronary Heart Disease Rates in Two Contrasting California Populations." In *Journal of Nutrition, Health and Aging* 9, no. 1 (January 2005).

———. *Diet, Life Expectancy, and Chronic Disease: Studies of Seventh-day Adventists and Other Vegetarians.* Oxford University Press, 2004.

———. "Vegetarian Diets: What Do We Know of Their Effects on Common Chronic Diseases?" In *American Journal of Clinical Nutrition* 89, no. 5 (March 2009).

Fraser, G. E., and D. J. Shavlik. "Ten Years of Life: Is It a Matter of Choice?" In *JAMA Internal Medicine* 161, no. 13 (2001).

Ros, E., L. C. Tapsell, and J. Sabaté. "Nuts and Berries for Heart Health." In *Current Atherosclerosis Reports* 12, no. 6 (November 2010).

Sabaté, J., et al. "Effects of Walnuts on Serum Lipid Levels and Blood Pressure in Normal Men." In *New England Journal of Medicine* 328 (March 1993).

Singh, P. N., J. Sabaté, and G. E. Fraser. "Does Low Meat Consumption Increase Life Expectancy in Humans?" In *American Journal of Clinical Nutrition* 78, 3 supplement (September 2003).

Tonstad, S., et al. "Vegetarian Diets and Incidence of Diabetes in the Adventist Health Study-2." In *Nutrition, Metabolism, and Cardiovascular Disease* 23, no. 4 (April 2013).

**CHAPTER 4: IKARIA**

Buettner, Dan. "The Island Where People Forget to Die." In *The New York Times Magazine,* October 24, 2012.

Georgirenes, Joseph. *A Description of the Present State of Samos, Nicaria, Patmos and Mount Athos.* London, July 14, 1677.

Legrand, Romain, et al. "Description of Lifestyle, Including Social Life, Diet and Physical Activity, of People ≥90 years Living in Ikaria, a Longevity Blue Zone." In *International Journal of Environmental Research and Public Health* 18, no. 12 (June 2021).

Panagiotakos, D. B., et al. "Sociodemographic and Lifestyle Statistics of Oldest Old People (> 80 Years) Living in Ikaria Island: The Ikaria Study." In *Cardiology Research and Practice,* 2011 (February 2011).

Tyrovolas, S., and D. B. Panagiotakos. "The Role of the Mediterranean Type of Diet on the Development of Cancer and Cardiovascular Disease in the Elderly: A Systematic Review." In *Maturitas* 65, no. 2 (February 2010).

**CHAPTER 5: OKINAWA**

Akisaka, M., et al. "Energy and Nutrient Intakes of Okinawan Centenarians." In *Journal of Nutritional Science and Vitaminology* 42, no. 3 (June 1996).

Rizza, W., N., Veronese, and L. Fontana. "What Are the Roles of Caloric Restriction and Diet Quality in Promoting Healthy Longevity." In *Ageing Research Reviews* 13 (January 2014).

Suzuki, M., D. C. Willcox, and B. J. Willcox. "The Historical Context of Okinawan Longevity: Influence of the United States and Mainland Japan." In *Okinawan Journal of American Studies,* 2007.

Willcox, B. J., D. C. Willcox, and M. Suzuki. *The Okinawa Program: Learn the Secrets to Healthy Longevity.* Three Rivers Press, 2001.

Willcox, B. J, D. C. Willcox, H. Todoriki, et al. "Caloric Restriction, the Traditional Okinawan Diet, and Healthy Aging: The Diet of the World's Longest-Lived People and Its Potential Impact on Morbidity and Lifespan." In *Annals of the New York Academy of Sciences* 1114 (October 2007).

**CHAPTER 6: SINGAPORE**

*Census of Population 2020: Statistical Release 1; Demographic Characteristics, Education, Language and Religion.* Singapore Department of Statistics, 2021.

**CHAPTER 7: THE POWER 9**

Cristakis, N. A., and J. H. Fowler. "The Spread of Obesity in a Large Social Network Over 32 Years." In *New England Journal of Medicine* 357 (July 2007).

Hummer, R.A., et al. "Religious Involvement and U.S. Adult Mortality." In *Demography* 36, no. 2 (May 1999).

**CHAPTER 8: THE BLUE ZONES FOOD GUIDELINES**

Pratt, S., and K. Matthews. *Superfoods Rx: Fourteen Foods That Will Change Your Life.* Harper, 2004.

**CHAPTER 9: CREATE YOUR BLUE ZONE**

Chen, K. W., et al., "Meditative Therapies for Reducing Anxiety: A Systematic Review and Meta-Analysis of Randomized Controlled Trials." In *Depression and Anxiety* 29, no. 7 (July 2012).

Darmadi-Blackberry, I., et al. "Legumes: The Most Important Dietary Predictor of Survival in Older People of Different Ethnicities." In *Asia Pacific Journal of Clinical Nutrition* 13, no. 2 (June 2004).

Ferrara, G., et al. "A Focused Review of Smartphone Diet-Tracking Apps: Usability, Functionality, Coherence With Behavior Change Theory, and Comparative Validity of Nutrient Intake and Energy Estimates." In *JMIR mHealth and uHealth* 7, no. 5 (May 2019).

LaRose, J. G., et al., "Frequency of Self-weighing and Weight Loss Outcomes Within a Brief Lifestyle Intervention Targeting Emerging Adults." In *Obesity Science and Practice* 2, no. 1 (March 2016).

Wansink, Brian. *Mindless Eating: Why We Eat More Than We Think.* Bantam Books, 2006.

Worley, S. L. "The Extraordinary Importance of Sleep: The Detrimental Effects of Inadequate Sleep on Health and Public Safety Drive an Explosion of Sleep Research." In *Pharmacy and Therapeutics* 43, no. 12 (2018).

Cover, Mark Thiessen/National Geographic; back cover, David McLain; 2–3, Andrea Frazzetta/National Geographic Image Collection; 4–6, David McLain; 9, David Sutherland/Alamy Stock Photo; 10, gianluigibec/Alamy Stock Photo; 13, David McLain; 14, Gen Umekita/Getty Images; 16–9, Gianluca Colla/National Geographic Image Collection; 20–1, Roslan Rahman/AFP via Getty Images; 22–3, David McLain; 26–7, Andrea Frazzetta/National Geographic Image Collection; 28–31, David McLain; 32, David McLain/National Geographic Image Collection; 33, Steffen Rothammel/mauritius images GmbH/Alamy Stock Photo; 34–5, Randy Olson/National Geographic Image Collection; 36 (UP LE), Hans-Peter Huber/Huber/eStock Photo; 36 (UP RT), Herby Meseritsch/Adobe Stock; 36 (LO), Ulrich Reichel/imageBROKER/Alamy Stock Photo; 37, Bruno Morandi/Sime/eStock Photo; 38 (UP), Olimpio Fantuz/Sime/eStock Photo; 38 (LO), Y. Levy/Alamy Stock Photo; 39, Gianluca Colla/National Geographic Image Collection; 40–1, Andrea Frazzetta/National Geographic Image Collection; 42, Alessandro Addis/Sime/eStock Photo; 43, David McLain; 44, Enrico Spanu/REDA&CO/Universal Images Group via Getty Images; 45, Bruno Morandi/Sime/eStock Photo; 46–7, Remi Benali/National Geographic Image Collection; 48, Nataša Mandić/Stocksy; 49, Joel Douillet/Alamy Stock Photo; 50–1, Gianluca Colla/National Geographic Image Collection; 53, Enrico Spanu/REDA&CO/Universal Images Group via Getty Images; 54–5, Gianluca Colla/National Geographic Image Collection; 56, David McLain; 58, Nicole Franco/National Geographic Image Collection; 59, Alexander Solorzano/Getty Images; 60–1, Gianluca Colla/National Geographic Image Collection; 62–3, David McLain; 64, Gianluca Colla/National Geographic Image Collection; 65 (UP and LO LE), David McLain; 65 (LO RT), Gianluca Colla/National Geographic Image Collection; 66, Gianluca Colla/National Geographic Image Collection; 67 (UP and LO), David McLain; 68–9, Nicole Franco/National Geographic Image Collection; 70–1, David McLain; 72, Nicole Franco/National Geographic Image Collection; 73, David McLain; 74–5, Gianluca Colla/National Geographic Image Collection; 76 (UP and LO), David McLain; 77, Matthieu Paley/National Geographic Image Collection; 78, David McLain; 79, Gianluca Colla/National Geographic Image Collection; 80, James L. Peacock/Alamy Stock Photo; 81, Nicole Franco/National Geographic Image Collection; 82–3 (UP LE and UP RT), David McLain; 83 (LO), Gianluca Colla/National Geographic Image Collection; 84–5, Travelstoxphoto/Getty Images; 87–9, Nicole Franco/National Geographic Image Collection; 90–4, David McLain; 95, Nicole Franco/National Geographic Image Collection; 96–7, David McLain; 98 (UP LE), Joseph Philipson; 98 (UP RT and LO)–100, David McLain; 101, Nicole Franco/National Geographic Image Collection; 102–4, David McLain; 105, David McLain/National Geographic Image Collection; 106–13, David McLain; 114, Joseph Philipson; 115, David McLain; 116–7, Travis Duran/EyeEm/Getty Images; 119, David McLain; 120–1, Johanna Huber/Sime/eStock Photo; 122–4, David McLain; 125, Percy Ryall/Alamy Stock Photo; 126, Gabriele Croppi/Sime/eStock Photo; 127–9, David McLain; 130, Gianluca Colla/National Geographic Image Collection; 131 (UP and LO RT), David McLain; 131 (LO LE), Ferruccio Carassale/Sime/eStock Photo; 132 (UP), Cavan Images/Getty Images; 132 (LO), David McLain; 133, Gianluca Colla/National Geographic Image Collection; 134–5, David McLain; 136, Gianluca Colla/National Geographic Image Collection; 137, David McLain; 138, Gianluca Colla/National Geographic Image Collection; 139, David McLain; 140, Gabriele Croppi/Sime/eStock Photo; 141 (UP), Gianluca Colla/National Geographic Image Collection; 141 (LO), David McLain; 142–3, Gianluca Colla/National Geographic Image Collection; 144, Sophie McAulay/Alamy Stock Photo; 145–7, David McLain; 149, Gianluca Colla/National Geographic Image Collection; 150–2, David McLain/National Geographic Image Collection; 154, David McLain; 155, Aflo Relax/Masterfile; 156, David McLain/National Geographic Image Collection; 157, David McLain; 158–9, Gianluca Colla/National Geographic Image Collection; 160 (UP LE), funkyfood London—Paul Williams/Alamy Stock Photo; 160 (UP RT), Ian Trower/robertharding; 160 (LO), Gianluca Colla/National Geographic Image Collection;

Dan Buettner is the founder of Blue Zones, an organization that helps Americans live longer, healthier, happier lives. His groundbreaking work on longevity led to his 2005 *National Geographic* cover story "The Secrets of Long Life" and four national best-sellers: *The Blue Zones, Thrive, The Blue Zones Solution,* and the number one *New York Times* best-seller *The Blue Zones Kitchen*. He is also the author of *The Blue Zones American Kitchen* and *The Blue Zones of Happiness.* He lives in Miami, Florida. Find him on Instagram (@danbuettner) and at danbuettner.com.

Blue Zones employs evidence-based ways to help people live longer, better. Beginning in 2004, Dan Buettner teamed with *National Geographic* and the National Institute on Aging to identify pockets around the world where people lived measurably better, longer lives. After locating the world's blue zones, Buettner took teams of scientists to each location to pinpoint lifestyle characteristics that might explain the unusual longevity. The original research and findings were released in Buettner's best-selling books *The Blue Zones, The Blue Zones Solution, Thrive*, and *The Blue Zones of Happiness.*

In 2009, Buettner and Blue Zones worked in partnerships with AARP and the United Health Foundation to apply the Blue Zones principles to Albert Lea, Minnesota. It was a "stunning success" and formed the blueprint for the Blue Zones Project, which has since expanded to more than 70 communities across the United States, impacting millions of people. This groundbreaking initiative has occasioned double-digit drops in obesity, smoking, and body mass index.

Learn more about the Blue Zones on Facebook (facebook.com/BlueZones), Twitter (@BlueZones), and Instagram (@BlueZones), and at bluezones.com.

National Geographic Partners, LLC
1145 17th Street NW
Washington, DC 20036-4688 USA

Get closer to National Geographic Explorers and photographers, and connect with our global community. Join us today at nationalgeographic.org/joinus

For rights or permissions inquiries, please contact National Geographic Books Subsidiary Rights: bookrights@natgeo.com

ISBN: 978-1-4262-2347-1

Printed in the United States of America

23/WOR/1

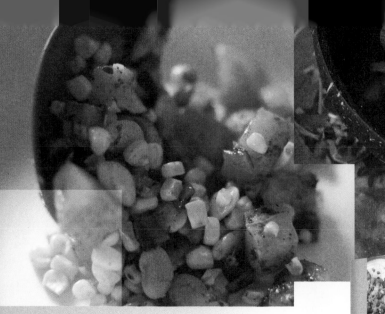

# 100 RECIPES TO EAT TO LIVE TO 100

*The Blue Zones American Kitchen* uncovers the traditional roots of plant-forward cuisine in the United States. In 100 tasty recipes, Dan Buettner showcases the regions and cultures that have shaped America's healthiest food landscapes. Along the way, he illuminates both traditional and revolutionary ideas in vegetarian food with recipes from chefs such as James Beard Award winner James Wayman, the "Gullah Chef" Bill Green, and Mohawk chef Dave Smoke McCluskey.

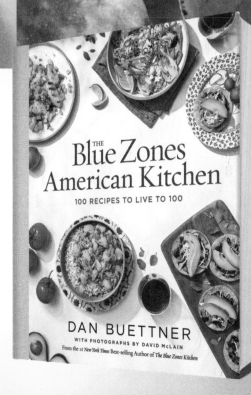

## LIVE LONGER, LIVE BETTER!

Discover these other books by Dan Buettner

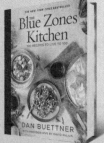
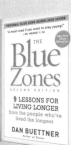
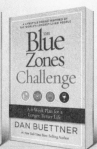
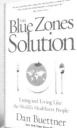
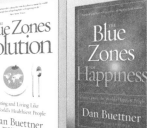
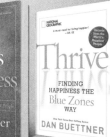